The Heart of Healing

Embracing Your Mindbody as the Path to Spiritual Awakening

MARY ANN WALLACE, MD

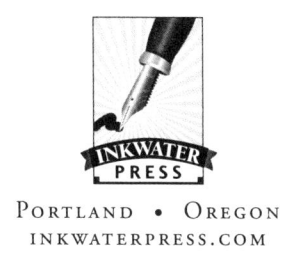

INKWATER PRESS

PORTLAND • OREGON
INKWATERPRESS.COM

Copyright © 2008 by Mary Ann Wallace, MD

Cover & interior designed by Tricia Sgrignoli/Positive Images

Cover photo © JupiterImages Corporation

All rights reserved. No part of this book may be reproduced or transmitted in any form or by any means whatsoever, including photocopying, recording or by any information storage and retrieval system, without written permission from the publisher and/or author. Contact Inkwater Press at 6750 SW Franklin Street, Suite A, Portland, OR 97223-2542. 503.968.6777

www.inkwaterpress.com

ISBN-10 1-59299-327-3
ISBN-13 978-1-59299-327-7

Publisher: Inkwater Press

Printed in the U.S.A.

All paper is acid free and meets all ANSI standards for archival quality paper.

CONTENTS

Acknowledgements ix
Foreword xi
Introduction xv

Chapter 1
  Your Body: the path to wholeness 1
    A wider view 3
    Waking up 8
    Your body as the anchor 13
    Overcoming resistance 15
    More about surrender 16

Chapter 2
  Emotion: energy in motion 18
    Constriction and the fight mentality 20
    Going beyond the story 23
    More about facing the fear 27
    A new way of being 30
    A balancing act 31

Chapter 3
  Mental Constructs: the blocks to wellness 33
    Recognizing your mental constructs 34
    Giving up the fight 37
    Shame and blame 38
    Working with complexes 40
    The larger picture 42

Chapter 4
Relationships: the field of play 44
- A dance of polarities 45
- Embracing relationship challenges 46
- Responsibility 51
- When the honeymoon ends 52
- Surrender 53

Chapter 5
Forgiveness: the foundation 55
- The path to forgiveness 55
- Forgiveness as healing 59

Chapter 6
Love: the heart of the matter 61
- Impediments to the awareness of love 62
- Romantic love 67

Chapter 7
Peace: your essential state 70
- Mental constructs as obstacles to peace 72
- Finding the peace within 74
- Peace meditation 77

Chapter 8
Soul: the portal to peace 79
- Pain as an access point 80
- Humans as the paradox 81
- Your soul's purpose 82

Chapter 9
Returning home: the dance 84

Appendix
Mindbody therapeutic techniques 91
- Breathwork 93
- Meditation 95
- What to expect when you begin meditating 97
- Meditative journaling 100

Imagery	103
Types of imagery	104
Goal of imagery therapies	107
Dreamwork	107
Working with the energy body	111
Endnotes	113
About the Author	117

ACKNOWLEDGEMENTS

This book has been a collaborative effort in its making.

My heartfelt gratitude goes to my editor and friend, Marie Oliver. From the very beginning, Marie believed in this project, and was able to take hours of the free flow of transcription, and transform it into readable prose. Her diligence often kept me on task when I may have more gladly stayed meditating.

My friends and readers: Jane Megard, Mike May, Rhonda Simpson, Linda Gelbrich, Susan Jewell-Larsen and Dan Benor all gave me invaluable feedback. I want to especially thank Dan Benor for editorial comments that added greatly to the final book.

Kristina Schnell, my beloved niece, took my photo for the insert.

And many, many people offered support and encouragement to "write the book". Larry Willits, Peg Mayo, Lani Maren, Tony Sedgman, Nick Wallace are but a few. In listing these, I leave out many.

We are all part of this effort. Thank you.

FOREWORD

*I*t is a pleasure and an honor to write these few words as foreword to The Heart of Healing. I have known Dr. Mary Ann Wallace for six years as a colleague and friend and have enormous admiration for her knowledge, wisdom and work. More than anything, though, it is her presence that I find the most impressive. Let me share about all of these, to put this book in perspective.

Dr. Wallace is very knowledgeable in the areas of conventional medicine, which serves her well in her work as director of the wellness center that she founded, nurtured to its present maturity and directs with a firm but light hand that invites staff to show and grow their own initiative. Dr. Wallace also consults to the rest of the conventional hospital that is home to the Wellness Center.

Dr. Wallace is also familiar with a broad spectrum of complementary therapies. This enables her to recommend holistic treatments that people who are receiving conventional care at her hospital can add to their treatment plans. She has taken the time and care to explore who in her community can provide such therapies, so recommendations for holistic care can be offered for patients' consideration. Dr. Wallace's broad experience in making these referrals enables her to speak with the confidence of clinical experience in addition to that of her educated opinions.

Dr. Wallace has a wisdom that is well-rounded, including: understanding the basics of medical knowledge that explain illnesses and diseases within the conventional, allopathic medical model; understanding the wholistic spectrum of contributing factors (in body, emotions, mind, relationships and spirit) that may contribute to the development and treatment of these problems; a strong gift of pattern recognition that enables her quickly to grasp the essence of a problem and the interrelationships of its component parts, possible interventions and potential outcomes; and a strong intuition that guides her life and her work.

It is in her presence, however, that her greatest gift resides. Dr. Wallace holds a quiet space in which another person can rest. This enables people who are in her presence to feel that they are being held in unconditional love and acceptance, and are being invited to find that same space within themselves. This is one of the highest forms of healing. It is readily apparent from details she shares in this book that Dr. Wallace has worked on herself to clear the vessel through which her healing flows, (to be as open as possible to invite spiritual awareness and healing into her work with people, through this presence.) It is my belief that she also brings with her the benefits of work done in other lifetimes.

This book is about ways that our illnesses can invite us to look deeper into ourselves, and ways that we can transform the illness from a travail into an invitation to understand ourselves more deeply. A sign of good teachers is that their teachings are readily understandable. All of Dr. Wallace's attributes detailed above enable her to help patients grasp that which they need for their healing. In this book, Dr. Wallace's many experiences and explanations of this special quality of presence in her work have been boiled down to: "face, embrace, and allow space." Keeping these in mind, you will be able to see and understand the ways in which presence can become a part of your practice, too.

When you can be in that state of presence, you will find that your own work and life are much easier to live. You will be in a flow of energies and relationships with those around you, not feeling pressures to be doing so much to bring joy and healing into your world but rather allowing yourself and those around you to find that place of being in which you invite the joy to enter and healing to happen.

And then there's the 'S' word, spirituality. This is a sense of connection with something vastly greater than ourselves. This has been given many names, most of which have been used in various religious or other contexts and have acquired all sorts of baggage in nuances. Dr. Wallace also shares in this book ways in which she helps people to connect with this vital aspect of themselves, which can add many dimensions to healing.

With this introduction, I am pleased to turn you over to the capable, healing hands of Dr. Wallace.

Daniel J. Benor, MD, ABHM
Author of Healing Research, Volumes I-III

INTRODUCTION

Mindbody and energy medicine has become a way of life for me. I integrate these modalities in my practice on a daily basis and have created a thriving Integrative Medicine clinic in a fairly conservative medical system. It has been a long and interesting path to get to this place. I share with you here a collage of the many formative experiences I have had on my path to writing this book, to put in perspective what I write.

The first time I was exposed to energy medicine, I had no clue what was going on. I was working in a busy metropolitan hospital one night, filling in for the head nurse who was out sick. As I was running down the hall to catch two IVs before they went dry, I heard sobs coming from a room to my right. I remembered that the patient in that room was a 15-year-old girl who had been hospitalized the day before. Linda had been in a motor vehicle accident from which she sustained multiple fractures. She was lying flat on her back, immobilized by several different kinds of traction. While in the emergency room, she had learned she was pregnant. In that moment when I was running by her room, I was moved by a state that I now call compassion, although back then I simply knew I was having an unusual, out-of-time, internal experience that had no category in my mind. I seemed to be magnetically pulled into the room, wishing so much that I could do something for Linda. I could not give her any more morphine because I did not want to depress her breathing and risk pneumonia. Instead, I went around to the head of the bed and wove my hands through all the tubing and gently placed them on her head. Instantly, I felt as if I had been plugged into an electrical current. Streams of a prickly sensation coursed down my arms and I felt my body becoming very relaxed and warm. I stood mesmerized as I watched this current flow through me to her. I could see her body ripple with waves of relaxation, and she fell sound asleep.

I was in an altered state of mind for the rest of the evening. I knew something had happened, but I did not know what. I had never heard of such a thing. For a long time, I referred to the current that flowed through me to her as electricity, because I did not know what it was. I'm still not sure that we really know, but today we call it "energy." Whatever it is, it is activated when our physiology is moved by a deep state of compassion and complete openness.

Today, I think in terms of surrendering into the infinite wealth of love that is available to us all. When we are in that space, we tap into the flow of the life force from which we originate and to which we return. Accessing that space involves dropping all judgment, being completely present in the moment, and being moved by compassion.

A few years later, I was the program coordinator for a small county health department in Oregon. In that capacity, I had just come back from a home visit with a family of twelve on which I was doing an epidemiological survey for a diarrhea outbreak. I remember thinking that these people were all drinking the same water and living the same basic lifestyle, but even though they were exposed to the same amount of bacteria, some would get sick and some would not. "What is that about?" I wondered. "Yes, we have to take the varying immune systems into account, but what is that about?" That seed of awareness prompted me to go back to school for a master's degree in psychology. I wanted to understand what internal influences at the individual level might be affecting the biology. I also began training in Chinese medicine and the very powerful Jin Shin Do acupressure method, which helped me to make some important mental connections. The paradigm from which Chinese medicine has evolved fits what I have observed in life. Five thousand years ago, medical practitioners were not allowed to cut into people, so they did not use tissue-based descriptors. Wellness was defined by relationship to one's environment, family, and food. The training is fundamentally different from the Western training model. Although it was rigorous and I was immersed in it day and night, it was also very health-promoting for me personally. I lived with my teacher for a while, and I was the school within which I was learning.

I was exposed to the Native American culture from an early age; my father worked on an Indian reservation and was "taken in" by the tribe. My mother preferred the services of a local medicine man over modern medicine, and often treated our childhood ailments with herbs purchased from Andy. I have always felt a special affinity for the teachings I gained in those formative years. In my twenties and early thirties, I experienced and then facilitated numerous vision quests. During one of my most pivotal vision quests, I was fasting in solitude and being with nature when I noticed a flock of birds flying over. They were all turning at exactly the same time, and I found myself wondering where to draw the line between the seemingly individual birds, because the whole flock really appeared to be one flying organism. That experience changed my perception of the entire world. I suddenly understood that everything is like that – there is no separation. I was looking around and thinking, "Where do we draw the line? We arbitrarily draw a line and give it a name. But you could just as easily draw the line somewhere else. How do we separate things out?"

I had a buddy, Susan, in one of these solitary vision quests of four days with whom I checked in each morning and afternoon by leaving a symbol at a predetermined place. Soon after the experience with the flock of birds, I was watching a hawk and suddenly I felt myself merge with it, and I was looking down on Susan. I could see her very clearly, lying on her belly in her sleeping bag, writing in her journal. Then, just as quickly, I was back where I had been sitting, looking at a rock. When Susan and I met to walk back down the mountain, I asked her what she was doing on day three. She said, "Well, I spent a lot of time in my sleeping bag, writing. And it was the most amazing thing, there was this hawk overhead and I felt so in tune, like it was talking to me." I realized that was me.

I was introduced synchronistically to my first formal meditation teacher in 1980. In the early 1990s, after I had been meditating daily for many years, I began having terribly painful experiences every afternoon. I was working as an epidemiologist at the time, and every day around three o'clock my spine would get so hot I dripped with sweat. I could barely stand the touch of clothing on my body as I leaned back in my chair. At the same time, the walls of the room seemed to get wavy and not quite solid. In fact, nothing seemed solid. Concurrently, my dream life and my waking life became so fluid and intermixed I could not tell where one left off and the other began. I lost considerable weight, even though I was eating voraciously. I am now so grateful that I did not mention these experiences to people within the conventional system, because I'm sure I would have been put on medication or locked up or diagnosed with some dreadful condition. Instead, I lived with it—and the fear—in my solitude. At times I was certain I was hearing conversations in another part of the building, and the couple of times I checked my perception by going to the room where I thought the conversation was happening, my perceptions were confirmed. It was not uncommon at all for me to have a dream, then go into the office and walk right into the dream I had just had. I would feel confused, wondering, "Is this the dream or was the dream earlier?" I knew what was going to happen, because I had already experienced it—it was all de'ja vu.

Concurrently, my former mother-in-law, to whom I did not mention any of these happenings, sent me a book on kundalini, the spontaneous, transformative rising of energies up the spine. I read it all in one sitting, crying all the way through because I finally understood what was happening to me. The book precisely described my experience. This unexpected synchronistic gift gave me a language to explain my experience as "normal" within the parameters and framework of kundalini rising. With that information, I was able to selectively choose a wise person to talk to about it. He suggested some visualizations to help calm the energy a bit so I could function in my daily life. Many nonordinary events occurred during that time—it was a time of enormous opening and it led me to a new willingness to trust.

My career life has fluctuated back and forth between left-brained (epidemiologist) and right-brained (energy healer/counselor) modes. Events have propelled me from one career path to another, often rather suddenly. It was while at a conference in Denver in 1990—as an epidemiologist—that it first occurred to me to become a physician. Being an epidemiologist at that time was a left-brained relief from the rigors of teaching and healing work I had been engaged in for several years. I thought I was done with patient care. But as I sat in that conference hall listening to a lecture by a female physician, I was hit with the whole-body awareness that I could be a physician. When I got home, I went straight to the dean's office at the medical school to discuss the possibility. The next week, I was sitting in a physics class—the first of many pre-med requirements I needed to fulfill before admittance to medical school.

As a practicing physician, people came to me because they were suffering in some manner. At first, to address a case of strep throat, I could write a prescription for penicillin and send them out the door. But I would still wonder, "How is it that your immune system is so suppressed and you are such a young person and nobody else in your family has this condition?" I was frequently relieved when someone came in for something simple like having a wart burned off—almost everything else raised questions for me, especially chronic or painful conditions. I wanted to know, "What's going on with this person?" "What's the story behind this?"

While I carefully applied all of my medical knowledge to each person's problems, I soon found myself practicing medicine more as a healer than as a conventional doctor. Treating only the body was not enough. In keeping with my basic philosophy of searching for the deeper message – the underpinning and true cause of suffering – I started spending more time with people.

I found it extremely difficult just to write prescriptions for people when I knew that the story behind their situation was often the

xix

cause of their suffering. Increasingly, with patients who were receptive, I started asking leading questions such as "What do you think that's about?" or "How does this symptom or illness fit in with the rest of your life?". I "feel" undercurrents of energy patterns, using a sense we do not have a word for to "see" energy. Eventually I started inviting people explicitly for mindbody work, adding imagery, acupressure and energy work to my conventional practice.

My devotion to this practice makes sense to me as a physician who addresses the whole person, not just symptoms and diseases. This has led me to dedicate my life to teaching and writing on this subject. I believe this is the wave of the future rising in a groundswell of awareness in the present. It is what we long for—to be heard and understood, and to understand ourselves as a whole within which the pathology is trying to teach us something.

We need our healers to listen to us deeply enough, to help us remember who we really are. Mindbody medicine calls upon its practitioners to practice what we preach. Mindfulness, meditation, awareness of Presence is required for all the individuals in the room when healer and client come together under the auspices of this more wholistic paradigm. We are all trying to come back home to the sense of our innate wholeness. This book is meant to be a guide in that process.

The Heart of Healing

CHAPTER 1

Your Body: the path to wholeness

Jesus said, "I am the path." That is true for each of us. Our mind-body is the path we have chosen for awakening in this lifetime. In the several thousand year old Chinese medical tradition, the ruler or emperor of the "kingdom within" is called *Shen*, or "heart." Although *Shen* can refer to the biological heart, it also refers to a much greater aspect of being. *Shen* is called the emperor because it is believed to rule all facets of the self. It recognizes the inner and the outer as inseparable. To recognize *Shen* as the ruler of the kingdom means that we are not in conflict with life itself, the environment, or those around us. We have surrendered into the flow of life and we experience harmony within and without. *Shen* means that our heartbeat, our heart's willingness, and our individual will are aligned with that which is harmonious to life as it unfolds moment to moment.

In the Christian tradition, we talk about surrendering to God's will. Perhaps we might consider that God is not separate, but is in fact the breath of life itself. We describe it as a separate thing so we can talk about it, but it is not separate. It is God, or *Shen*, that we reflect in this life as human beings. *Shen* breathes as our own heartbeat. To surrender into *Shen* means we exist in trust and truth. It means we recognize that this moment, and every moment, is perfect as it is.

Surrendering to *Shen*, to God's will—or whatever terminology is useful to you—is the heart of healing. Through our health challenges, our bodies call us to surrender to a chosen path and allow that path to guide us. The Taoists have a useful phrase for this: *wu wei*. Strictly translated, *wu wei* means inaction, but it really means effortless living. It reflects the idea of "going with the flow"—not passively, but by engaging in natural and spontaneous action in the moment. It means taking action that flows naturally from being, unforced and without a self-serving agenda. It means surrendering to harmony, selflessness, generosity, and balance. When we are deficient in *Shen*, we experience doubt and insecurity and misery. We lack confidence and clarity, and we do not know where to turn. When we surrender to *Shen* as ruler of the kingdom, we surrender into confidence in the flow of life and ourselves as a part of that life. We meet life confidently and we fully engage with what is in front of us.

It is not uncommon, with a deficiency of Shen, to experience heart based fears. Sheila, a 64 year old woman, saw me after multiple emergency room visits for "heart pain" that turned out to be not heart related. After only one visit, we got to the core of her issue: she had such profound fear of dying from heart disease that every twinge of pain in the chest area was immediately translated into fear of death. Living with the anxiety was provoking a living hell for her; learning to strengthen a sense of herself in the here and now as fully alive - until death actually occurs – freed her from the recurrent emergency room visits.

True health is a spiritual endeavor. Every message coming through us as our physical experience offers something we can learn from. Our fears keep us confined to a box of comfortable activity that does not threaten our sense of safety too much. To fully realize and activate our capability requires surrendering the fear by which we define ourselves. In psychological or mythical terms, it means embracing our shadow. It means facing the dragons of our psyche. It means squaring off on the mental patterns that keep us restricted and constricted. It means we engage in a spiritual act by jumping over that threshold into asking questions of the heart. We ask questions like: "Why am I restricted?" "What facts do I hold as self-evident that require me to turn life against myself through this symptom or illness or disharmony in my life?" "Why do I believe I'm not worthy?" "How am I ingrained in a resonance of suffering?" "Where have I accepted suffering as my way of life?" These are primarily spiritual and psychological questions and they point to the actions and behaviors that dictate whether we experience health and wellness or disease. That is the true "mindbody connection." In actuality, no mindbody connection is required, because *there is no separation.*

As we surrender to *Shen*, we begin to redefine ourselves. We experience ourselves not as a personality or a body, but as points in time—an active energy participating in the flow of life. We no longer fear loss. Joy becomes the primary attribute of living completely in the state of *Shen*. It is the balanced place of heart that is our potential.

A WIDER VIEW

Today we see an alarming increase in disease states that result from the life force attacking and turning against itself. It is no surprise that the primary cause of death in both men and women today is heart disease. Heart disease occurs when clogged arteries cause the heart tissue to die from lack of oxygen and nutrients. Likewise, when we prioritize our work or another life function over relationship and over the importance of listening to our heart's passion, we experience a diminishing of self, a spiritual starvation or even a cutting off from the life blood of our higher selves. Ultimately, as humans, we stand in the amazing position of having the capacity to define our relationship with life in its many aspects. That's what it means to have free will. When we define ourselves in maladaptive ways, this will demonstrate in our experience of ourselves in life – and show up in our bodies as illness.

Metaphorically speaking, attending to the inner emotional framework could be seen as that lubricating force that is analogous to the blood that flows through our arteries. When those arteries are clogged—when we no longer attend to our relationships or our heart's desire—our life's blood gets clogged and can no longer nourish the heart that is central to our ongoing function as a human being. Research shows that suppressed anger predisposes to heart disease. Recent data supports the notion that elevated enzymes indicating an inflammatory state are a predominant feature in heart disease. Again thinking metaphorically, this adds another wrinkle of awareness when we couple that knowledge with data that correlates anger and stress with heart disease.

Autoimmune diseases are another prime example of the body attacking itself. Examples of these diseases include diabetes, rheumatoid arthritis, lupus, and many others. In each of these cases, the immune system misidentifies some part of the body as "foreign", and attacks it as a pathogen. Anorexia and other pathologies that have clear mental, emotional, and physical components are more obvious profound examples of self-abuse. At the risk of being too simplistic, it is not uncommon for individuals who suffer from anorexia to have grown up in situations where criticism was the norm. The sufferer's family may have tended toward a functional perfectionism and rigidity that lacks gentleness and does not accept the individual's beauty, perspective, perception, identity, and uniqueness. In reaction, the subconscious mind turns against itself through self-induced starvation. Similarly, it is common for individuals who suffer from rheumatoid arthritis to have some held-in bitterness, often with angers accumulated that are reflected in joint inflammation. These illnesses are opportunities—wake-up calls—that invite those who suffer to reflect within themselves. When we ask ourselves the question of "what am I trying to tell myself?" free of judgment or blame, we open the door to greater self understanding.

Please do not blame yourself or anybody else for your illness—that just creates a whole new set of problems. Nobody has done anything wrong. "New age" thinking often wants to put old wine in new wine skins so to speak, so you end up with a guilt-laden sense that might be reflected in thoughts such as, "What did I do wrong to bring cancer on me?" or even worse, "What did *you* do wrong to bring cancer on *you*?" Let go of guilt and blame —you do not need it. Rage or blame against the self is not much different than rage against someone else. In taking responsibility for your health, it is important to release any sense of blame whatsoever. Far from being one more pathway for harshness against yourself, searching within for the cause of illness can provide a gentle pathway of forgiveness and self-acceptance. Instead of blaming yourself when you are having an experience in your body, rest in the resonance of the experience as deeply as you can. Open your heart, surrender, and ask, "What is this? What can I learn here?" Surrender as much as you can into the frequency and the vibration of the experience. It is vitally important that you drop judgment. Judgment contextualizes your experience and wraps a negative meaning around it, and then you have so much wrapping around the whole thing you forget the present moment. You have forgotten that each moment contains infinite possibility because you are living the entrapments of this contextualized situation.

Cancer reflects an immune system that makes poor choices. It actually turns off the protective processes that are congruent with the innate life force and allows destructive forces to take over. On the manifest level, you may observe this in the poor decisions and choices you may make on a day-to-day basis regarding food consumption, activities, and the way your emotional currency is spent. On the physical level, it shows up as the immune system not recognizing those maladaptive cells that have gone awry as problematic and therefore allowing their rampant proliferation as the disease we call "cancer".

Taking the earth metaphor a step further, we could apply the same terms used to describe cancer to describe our behavior on the planet. Imagine that you are far removed from the earth and looking back at it. You might see it as a living organism, and it would be obvious that the ravaging and destructive force of cancer is prevalent. You would see gaping holes where destruction has occurred, such as abandoned mines or treeless, eroded hillsides. You would see humanity clinging onto the earth's surface, clustered in gross, tumorlike formations. And surrounding these large growths you would see the countless damaging effects of mistreating our planet. Earth's polluted waters are analogous to our clogged arteries.

In actuality, this is more than a metaphor. Our lives poetically reflect the choices that humanity is making. These choices are profoundly reflected both outside and inside ourselves. The earth's suffering is palpable—we can imagine that her reaction is akin to the fury of anyone who has been so dishonored.

We humans have an enormous egocentricity about ourselves, presuming to be the center of the universe. It is time for us to recognize that everything happening in our biology is reflected in the earth and in our relationships, and adapt ourselves to that recognition. We are not separate from the earth and we know ourselves within the context of relationships. Statements we can make about our relationships are true in our bodies, and vice versa. It is no secret that relationships make a profound difference in survival rates among people with chronic diseases such as cancer, heart disease, and so on. Study after study demonstrates the protective effects of a healthy social support system to such maladies as heart attacks and depression. Likewise, emotional states such as hostility directly impact the incidence, prevalence, and outcomes of certain diseases states such as heart disease. When we recognize this, we embrace a different paradigm of relating, acting, and behaving. Rather than simplistically thinking of our choices in self centered ways, we begin to recognize how profound and influential each choice really is.

It is not uncommon for diseases to be carried forward generation to generation through genetics, lifestyle choices, and so forth. Likewise, emotional issues are carried forward generation to generation. So it is worthwhile to reflect upon our family's heritage as it pertains to disease states or health challenges. When we recognize that a simple genetic code that makes us susceptible to certain diseases can also reflect deeper soul issues, we begin to uncover the potential for literally changing humanity. Each person has the capacity to change the entire movement of life flowing through his or her family of origin. When we embrace and deal with the issues that face us as exactly what needs to be addressed in our lifetime, we also make a change in our entire family lifestream.

We must begin to embrace the notion that relationship itself is the fundamental factor wherein we will find help and define ourselves in healthy ways. In the past two decades we have increasingly identified certain situations as codependent and pathologic, and this is an important recognition. When we compromise our core values to aid and abet another's addictions we do great harm to all involved. Unfortunately, we can go overboard the other way and believe that the answer is to be strongly individualistic. Our wisdom tells us that only within ourselves will we find the answer. That is true, but it is true in a more holistic sense. The entire body's information is contained as a holograph within one DNA strand. In similar fashion all the information that is played out in our lives can be found contained within the self. However, it is enacted and played out in the choices we make *in the context of relationship*—the relationship between ourselves and others, the relationship between ourselves and the earth, the relationship between ourselves and work, and every other relationship we can possibly imagine. In the context of relationship, we can remember and recall the state of wellness of which we are capable. We call back from the darkness those parts of ourselves we have forgotten or denied.

We must define our relationship with the earth in a healthy way, recognizing that we are *of the earth*. The air in our lungs is that of the environment around us, our bodies are composed of the elements of this very earth we inhabit. We simply must become responsible and recognize ourselves less egocentrically—it is essential for our survival. The notion of engaging in battle with the *source of our life*, of conquering the earth, is ridiculous. The war mentality that is reflected in the battle on pathogens is in fact a nihilistic approach that eventually will bring about destruction of the earth that feeds us and sustains us—the earth from which we come and to which we return. Striving only to kill – bacteria inside, "pests" outside – creates a constant influx of poison that impacts our body and the earth in like fashion.

We must look at every facet of life with deep reverence. Every molecule of form that shows up in our experience brings us an opportunity to embrace life with love, compassion, and respect. If we do that, we will turn within ourselves with that same deep love and compassion.

WAKING UP

"Waking up" is the phrase used in many spiritual disciplines to describe the process by which we remember our true nature. Most spiritual disciplines have some variation of what this true nature looks and feels like. In describing the spiritually awakened state, we might hear adjectives like loving, kind, and generous. Unfortunately, sometimes we circumvent our real awakening by adopting a stance that we believe projects those adjectives instead of doing the painful work that is necessary to truly embody them. For example, in an effort to demonstrate the image of being awakened, we might paste onto ourselves a "nice guy" image or a "sweet girl" image, and so forth. That, of course, is simply the outermost layer of pretense, but we can seduce ourselves into believing that it reflects reality and that we are awakened. We put up great defenses against anyone revealing what is still hidden within our deep layers of fear. We cover up our most deeply held belief that at our core we are not okay.

The awakening process can be exceptionally painful and chaotic. There is no way around that. Imagine that you have frozen fingers from having been outside in the cold too long. They go numb and you might even almost forget where they are because you cannot feel them. When you come inside and warm up, you experience pain when your fingers begin to awaken—it is a remarkably uncomfortable sensation. Waking up from spiritual slumber is like that, but it lasts much longer and goes much deeper.

We all have deep psychic scars. Whether one believes in karma, or simply traces the impact of messages we incorporate as reality in our growing up process, we all have internal spaces in which we perceive some part of ourselves or others as "not OK". As humans, we share a fundamental flaw in our thinking and we keep it going by unconsciously conspiring with each other in the cover-up. To the extent that we believe ourselves to be separate from the whole of life, we are miserable. Advertising is effective by activating the terrible discomfort of these deeply nested anxieties. We are seduced into believing that we are not okay unless this, unless that, or unless something else—we tend to focus on the image. Awakening begins when you develop a fundamental honesty about the crack in your self-image—that which you most do not want to see. *Anything* that makes you feel uncomfortable can be a clue that you are on the track of waking up to some old scar. Does that mean you seek out pain? Of course not. In fact, you might find yourself getting caught in the trap of putting yourself in painful situations where you have to persevere, thereby "proving" to yourself that you are worthy of the challenge. That is a false sense of waking up. However, it can be a step along the way. If the pain gets severe enough, one day you will wake up to the fact that you do not need it anymore. At some point, we all get to that place.

The thawing out process can be gradual or it can come about suddenly as the result of a crisis. It does not matter how you get there. What matters is that at some point you experience a sense of emotional nakedness. You begin to be self-revealing about the discomfort and the stuff that brings you shame. Shame is a hot marker—it is a clue that you need to look deeper. In the Garden of Eden myth[1], Adam and Eve needed to cover themselves because of shame, and their final uncovering still needs to happen. The archetype of this pattern lives within every person in some way. Whether explained as the psychological imprinting of childhood experiences, karma or the original sin, there lives within every person that place in which he or she feels "not good enough". The paradox is that in that final revealing, in the unmasking of that place where you experience your greatest shame, you will discover to your amazement and awe a profound sense of innocence. You can see the innocence within it, like you might see the innocence in a baby's nudity. You discover an astounding sense of loving kindness, sweetness, openness, and the transcendence of fear you acquire through the hard work of getting there. Frankly, anything short of that is bravado and is simply covering up whatever you are still hiding from yourself and others.

There are several identifiable steps to awakening.

First, you develop a genuine desire to know the truth, and that desire is greater than any other desire. It burns greater than your desire to appear in any particular way, including appearing spiritual. When your authentic desire to wake up to the truth is greater than your desire to appear spiritual, you have taken a major step on the path.

Second, you develop a desire to be so deeply truthful that you are willing to endure whatever pain, embarrassment, or circumstances arise on your path. The Biblical story of Job[2] reflects this willingness. In that story you see the severe pain that Job endures because he loves God, which really means he loves the unvarnished truth.

The second part of the path can take any length of time, so the third step is developing the willingness for it to take however long it takes for the truth to reveal itself. It is the surrender step.

Surrender has so many definitions and connotations that many people are confused by what is meant by it. Spiritual surrender does not mean letting go of anything that is ultimately valuable or precious to you. It does not mean giving yourself up to another person or anything at all outside yourself. It does not mean inducing suffering as a statement of worthiness. For example, if you have a sense of a God that is outside you, you might share a notion that has evolved throughout the ages that to surrender requires some self-abnegation or self-depreciation. Untold suffering has happened to humanity in the name of that sort of surrender. Many religious dogmas, for instance, hold that women are inferior simply by rote of their gender. The pain inflicted – and supported – in the name of this inequity runs deep in the psyches of many women today.

True surrender does not mean giving up anything except falsehoods. It simply means letting go of the restrictions and constrictions. True surrender is allowing yourself to be completely open to whatever is happening in any particular moment. You do not need to "figure out" what you need to let go of today. Let it all go. Getting in the head, sorting through details, weighing pros and cons, going around in mental circles, all are methods of increasing the inner tension that keeps you from just being fully here – right now – with what is in front of you. It is only by feeling the full impact of this moment that one actually has the necessary information to make an "informed' decision.

As long as you have a timeline, you are still seeking to control the process of awakening. In this third phase, you become willing to endure whatever arises and allow it to take however long it takes to pass. Real freedom comes from this surrender, because in a sense you evaporate the need to achieve. Almost every success formula in the books these days stresses achieving a goal by a certain time, and we are admonished that if we do not establish those parameters, we do not know whether or not we have succeeded. We all have day planners, right? That is part of our goal-oriented culture. In this endeavor you must trash the timeline and be willing to engage in a process *no matter how long it takes.*

True surrender naturally facilitates humility. Authentic humility requires admitting that you do not know what is required. You do not know how long it is going to take, you do not know what the end will look like, you do not know what it feels like, and you do not claim to know before you do. Ironically, once you get closer to that goal of knowing, you become less inclined to claim that you know anything at all. So the fourth step, authentic humility, means being willing to stand in the space of "I don't know." Again, this is not pseudo-humility where you cast up your eyes saying, "I really don't know, God is in charge here" in a syrupy way that makes everyone around you pretty sure there is a one-upmanship going on. We are so trained to want to know, to need to know, that it gets tricky. We think, "Ah, I've got it, I know what to do. I can say I don't know!" Catch the irony in that. But be gentle with yourself—at least you are a bit more on track. You will learn that authentic "not knowing" reveals a whole new layer of nakedness.

The fifth step is a willingness to take what is in front of you and recognize it as the path and the only path available to you. To the extent that we are searching for the "right" path, we are missing the boat. Perhaps we are searching for the "right" teacher, the "right" teaching, the "right" wisdom to help us wake up. That then becomes your path because that is what is in front of you—your own inquisitive impatience. Let the impatience be your path. Enter deeply into the phenomenon of your experience *right where you are*. What does that impatience feel like in your body?

This step is where you develop a finely tuned awareness of your mindbody. Mindfulness meditation practices like *vipassana*[3] are extremely helpful. You can choose sitting meditation or walking meditation, it does not matter so long as the method is designed to facilitate becoming cognizant of what is going on inside you at any given time. See the Appendix for an overview of some popular practices. You can get started now as you read this book. Choose a practice that helps you to become more finely tuned to your emotional state and how you experience it physically. You will begin to embrace the truth of the experience you are having *in the moment you are having it,* and that is a unique kind of nakedness. Coupled with that are all the aforementioned steps wherein you remain honest, unapologetic and accepting. You just are where you are. As you develop more acuity with this step, you begin to recognize that all these steps are fluctuating and inter-related states of being that eventually proceed without making a conscious effort.

Step five transitions automatically into a deep-seated trust, which is step six. You do not do anything to make this step happen—it evolves naturally. When you have deeply surrendered, you develop an abiding trust that every sensation, every emotion, and every experience you have will automatically transition. There is nothing you can do and nothing you have to do. By now, you know you are not in control and you no longer make effort to be in control because you know better. You no longer *need* to have control because you trust, and you trust because you know that you are not in control! Paradox becomes the rule of the game. You no longer rely on human roles to accomplish things.

At this point, you gain trust in a bigger picture that defies definition. Here we move to a place where words no longer suffice to describe the experience. Words are pointers that facilitate a certain resonance beyond which the being surrenders and no longer has the words to explain the experience. Words are simply like door posts marking the doorway. You move beyond the three-dimensional plane and you experience a magnetic pull to a center around which you and all beings originate. All sensations change. Once you pass through that doorway and you come back down off the mountain, life is different. It is different because you are awake.

YOUR BODY AS THE ANCHOR

You forget that you are spirit. Pay attention. Look how temporary this life is that you call your physical life. Your body is the path that is given to you to facilitate your awakening to that remembering. Your physical experience *is what is*. Your body is not only the path, it also serves as the anchor—the reality base from which and with which you operate in the world. It continually demonstrates the inner reflections that are playing out in your life. If you ever have a question as to your inner workings, you can refer to the body's reality for a "check in." In the spiritual trek, it is too easy to become disassociated and live in your head. But physical existence is nothing to escape—it is the path. Coming back to the body again and again anchors you in the here and now, in the real situations in which you find yourself. Every event, including and most particularly the events of your body such as disease or illness, are your path to awakening. *Every phenomenon that occurs in your body is a wake-up call.*

Recognize the gift of the present moment as exactly where you need to be. You are having a continual experience, and that experience is your body. The farther outside yourself you get, the more you remove yourself from the real issue. In psychology we use words like projection, in religion we call it blame—it does not matter what you call it—anything that has all your energy looking outward is missing the point. Instead of wiping the mirror, constantly trying to get the smudge off your face, stop. Feel your body, your experience, and rest in that. Many patients come to me with aggravation, saying things like, "Dr. Wallace, what can I do to get rid of this symptom? How can I get rid of my belly ache? What could be the problem here?" But it is not a problem, you see—it is an invitation.

Every nuance of your physical experience comes and goes. As you embrace all the details of life and living, it becomes much easier to rest in the sense of spaciousness simultaneous to having the experience. As the Buddha teaches, interpreting your experience as suffering ceases. To the extent that you accept all your experience as it is and live in the present moment—knowing that it is constantly changing—you realize that in fact you are that spaciousness Itself. Then the breath in and the breath out becomes simply a nuance playing across the harp of the life experience. You just notice, and see what is there. You watch it, notice it, and smile—a lot! This sense of peaceful acceptance is not something you paste on because Buddha or some spiritual writer said so—you know it to be a fact because you have experienced it.

In the 1940s, psychologist Abraham Maslow gave us a model he called the hierarchy of needs.[4] This concept is also reflected in the ancient Hindu chakra[5] system. The basic idea here is that if we are functioning on a survival basis, it is difficult to open our minds and hearts to higher order needs. Although this is true on some level, it is also precisely through our deepest sorrow and pain that we are most ripe to awaken to our highest spiritual potential. This is reflected, for example, in India, where a country that houses incredible poverty embodies such a deep spiritual knowing. As mentioned earlier, it is also reflected in the yin yang symbol, where the darkest part contains the seed of light. We hear it in Christian language through reference to the "dark night of the soul." So wherever you are, whatever unmet needs you perceive you have, the invitation is to recognize that your suffering contains the seed of potential awakening. No exceptions. Any form of suffering contains that seed. And the part of you that makes excuses, that wants to be distracted from doing the work because you "don't have time," or "have to make a living," or "can't afford it," or whatever, is just another layer of the mind attempting to keep you trapped.

OVERCOMING RESISTANCE

Most people who are ill consciously want to get better. It is what we hold onto unconsciously or subconsciously that creates our problems. If, because of your illness, you have received attention that you were never able to acquire any other way, or if you have received financial compensation as a result of being ill, or if you have been able to avoid something because of your illness, you have a huge investment in it. Although the rewards might be obvious in the case of a financial settlement, at times the payoff is subtle and difficult to recognize. To give up attention, to lose a partner, to have to do life differently may be a tradeoff you are not willing to make for your health. When the payoff for being sick is greater than the potential advantage of wellness, no medicine in the world can cure you—and most assuredly your "inner pharmacy" will be locked up—until you make the decision at a deep level to be well.

To wake up, you must realize that you are not safe in this place of resistance, but you are actually trapped. Entrapment feels secure only because it is familiar. To risk going where you authentically have not gone before is scary beyond words, and beyond what most people are willing to do without a guide, assistance, or a major crisis to propel them into action. So health crises happen, loss happens—can that wake us up? Friendships happen; great love happens—is we ready to wake up? If so, we can begin to choose consciously. Maybe at times this looks like we are choosing pain, but we know there is method in the madness, and that method leads us to greater sanity and real, lasting health.

In this book, I explore the body as the path—the ways different disease states play out various chords of experience. In this exploration, it is important that you not take what I say as the absolute black-and-white truth for you. These are just suggestions to think about. What is most essential is that you surrender into the experience of *your* body at this moment in time. Let go into it, welcome it, embrace it, and ask, "What is this?" Drop your judgments. Stop seeking for an explanation for what you need to do differently to get rid of your experience. Instead, fling the door open, invite it in and say, "Ah, long lost friend! What are you here to tell me now?" With that attitude, it all gets easier. At some point, you truly embrace all of yourself as an adventure, even the pain—especially the pain. Pain keeps us on the razor's edge so that we cannot help but pay attention. You must stop anesthetizing yourself. The more you numb yourself, the longer the journey will be.

MORE ABOUT SURRENDER

You know you are on track when you feel a greater sense of freedom. You feel enlivened and grateful, warm and happy. If you feel like you are suffering because you are surrendering to God and you need to be punished, you are stuck in an old mindset. Humanity is ready to evolve beyond that belief structure, as evidenced by some of the more narcissistic practices and efforts toward self-enjoyment we see today. This reflects a spiritual calling to allow life to be a pleasurable adventure, and ultimately signals a positive shift in awareness. However, true enjoyment will not be noticed or realized or appreciated until true surrender happens. Surrender is hard work because you have to engage and move through the terrific fear that comes up when you question your reality as you have known it. But it does not require you to injure yourself through further punishment.

Surrender is the mechanism whereby you bless the earth through the vehicle of your self. You contain within the fabric of your structure all elements of the earth that need the heart's blessing. The heart is strategically placed in the center of your chest, pumping your life's blood constantly to keep your body alive, moving the life throughout your body. Likewise, you can infuse with awareness the wisdom of love so that it penetrates through every cell, through every bit of tension, and emanates into the earth around you. This is the beating heart of wisdom. In the Buddhist meditation practice of Tonglen, you breathe into your heart every bit of pain you imagine, suspect, or encounter, and you breathe out love. When you rest in the center of your heart, you are completely protected. You are pain free of pain. *This is possible.* It does not mean you will not experience tragedies, but you will redefine them as invitations. You will be in a different kingdom then, a truly different state of affairs. It is as if you are in a parallel universe right here on planet earth, and you will be a beacon of light for those around you. It is recognizable and it is palpable.

CHAPTER 2

Emotion: energy in motion

Emotional wellness is a complex subject. Each of us has our own conditioning that tells us certain emotions are "good" and others are "bad." Well, here is the news: emotions are neither good nor bad. Emotions are simply energy moving through the body. Emotions are not something to be gotten rid of, judged, or analyzed.

Anger, for example, in its truest form is really an urge to express authentically in the world. It has a positive intention—it is trying to accomplish something for you. Anger occurs when your authentic expression becomes blocked because of your mental framework. Just like a dam that holds the water back, any blockage in your system causes energy to build up behind it. Emotion is quite a beautiful thing, because it creates an opportunity to awaken you from clinging to a mental construct from an old awareness.

Every act is done either with a purity of intention, without apology, and is legitimate in that moment or it is not. If it is not, energy will be retained in the system in some pathologic way that becomes a storyline and a theme song for your life. Every emotion you might term negative has a pure expression that is a normal expression of your true self. The experience of any negative emotion is a clue to what mental constructs may be awry. For example, pure fear energy can motivate and energize an instantaneous action that is a normal response in the face of being overwhelmed. But because of your conditioning, your busy mind takes over. You monitor your actions and reactions to conform to your beliefs, accepted roles, or societal expectations. In this way, the purity of the energy in response to a threat can be compromised, and can lead to a chronic headache or backache or other physical symptom.

People come to see me with pain, and as we release the pain through mindbody work, emotions inevitably start to come to the surface. As the emotions are released the storyline surfaces. Your body will always tell the truth of your perceptual framework. It will not lie to you. The story is not ultimate truth, but it is the truth you live and, until you do the work, it is all you know. In mindbody work, the answer is always to bring attention to that which is maladaptive—to that which is tight, tense, and painful. To the extent the current medical model focuses on dulling or deadening pain with one form or another of anesthesia, it is less than helpful. People have trouble when they cannot feel whatever their inner self is calling their attention to—the part that is hurting and wanting attention. Shutting away the evidence rather than examining it may provide temporary anesthesia from pain, does it does not allow for authentic, deep healing.

The obesity epidemic in this country is an example of this tendency to anesthetize ourselves. For instance, Frances* came to see me to deal with her obesity. Through our work together, she realized that every diet she had ever tried had worked. However, whenever she lost enough weight that she began to feel attractive and sexy, what came to the surface was her terror of attracting unwanted attention. It was much easier to cover it up quickly than to deal with the feelings that were so overwhelming in her body.

Western medicine agrees with Chinese medicine on this: over-expressed or under-expressed emotions take their toll on the body. For example, scientists have done some wonderful double-blind controlled studies that prove anger and hostility are directly correlated with heart attacks and high blood pressure. Inevitably,

---

* All names have been changed to protect the identity of my patients. However, their experiences have been preserved.

such over-expressed emotions lead to the decline of the overtaxed body. This is in keeping with the centuries old 5 elements theory of Chinese Medicine.

On the other hand, if you repress your emotions, your sense of vitality may eventually be suppressed to the point of depression. Thus, suffering from depression can be a clue that you may be repressing anger and not giving yourself permission to express what you need to express in the world. It takes a lot to keep that energy under wraps, and that causes depression. On the other hand, you may *over-express* emotions. If you are experiencing grief and you do not let yourself get down into the kernel of it and do the actual letting go process, you will deplete your energy over time.

We carry our emotions and the associated mind-talk with us wherever we go—whether we are alone or in company. A few years ago, for instance, I was walking to the store one beautiful spring day and I had just stepped off the sidewalk to cross the street when I suddenly became aware that I was feeling tense and had an abrasive internal dialogue going on. I thought, "You know, I'm carrying on an argument in my head, and there's nobody else here! Who am I arguing with?" Most of us have conversations like that going on in our head all the time. As those conversations are going on, our body is reacting *as if the situation we are focused on were actually happening*. We play the part of each character in the scene, and our muscles tense in response to whatever we are thinking. In other words, our physiology is correlated with the thoughts we hold about our life experience. This is a very powerful recognition.

CONSTRICTION AND THE FIGHT MENTALITY

True emotional wellness comes when you allow every single flavor of energy movement in the body, which means that every emotion must find its natural voice. When you begin to pay attention to your mental patterns, you will begin to notice a relationship between the thoughts you are thinking and the emotions you are carrying. Then you will begin to notice an interrelationship among your thoughts, your emotions, and your physical structure. For example, if you experience chronic fear or anger, your body will begin to reflect constriction, and the sensations associated with that constriction sooner or later can become pain. If you pay attention, your emotions can provide clues through your body to what is getting in the way of your free and authentic interaction with life. In fact, you possess the best biofeedback mechanism on the planet!

The quality of emotion or bodily sensation you experience in response to different life situations depends on your belief system. Problems arise when beliefs, and the resulting constriction, take over. Whatever your beliefs are, they typically reflect a recurring theme, and the storyline can be recognized in our cultural archetypes and myths. A first step in moving beyond the storyline is recognizing that you hold different elements of it *within the physical structure of your body.*

For example, Betty came to see me to try to figure out why her stomach was hurting. The first time she saw me, she came to get rid of the symptoms. She had had all the appropriate medical tests to rule out an organic cause – but the pain was very real. We worked with imagery and internal dialogue to welcome a deeper understanding of what the pain was about. On the second visit, she said the symptoms were getting worse, but what was coming out of the work was so rich that she cared less about the pain and more about what was behind the pain. She realized she was there to find out what her stomach was trying to tell her. She learned that she had literally *stuffed* painful and frightening emotions around serious abuse in her childhood. She experienced a holding back, a "stuckness" in her energy matrix. She had swallowed down her emotional pain and her stomach was bringing this to her attention.

This type of holding-in symptom is interesting, because it typically includes more than one dynamic. It might also reflect a fear of releasing or a fear of expressing. The unwillingness to express might imply that Betty is afraid of the ramifications of fully expressing herself because she fears some sort of loss or punishment if she connects with and releases her emotions.

Constrictions or barriers to a healthy energy flow show up as fear, guilt, shame, anger, and feelings of helplessness. At the core level, you may believe that it is not possible to get what you want—that the object of your desire is not available in the world or that you are not worthy of it even if it is available. You believe that you have done something wrong, or are so bad that you do not deserve to get what you want. If you do get what you want, you believe it will probably be taken from you, so you hold on tight. This is the real meaning of what Christians call "original sin." To be driven out of the Garden of Eden means that when you exclude yourself from the flow of infinite possibility by your own mental constructs, you block from your energy matrix a significant portion of those possibilities that are inherent within you. And you do that through your own thinking. The detection, dismantling and releasing of these blocks is an exciting aspect of mindbody therapy, one that unfolds in infinite variations that are unique to each person.

We in the Western world are particularly yang—we approach our health like warriors: "Get out the battleaxe, fight that pathogen! Win this battle! Fight that enemy!" We must learn to cultivate the yin aspect. We must surrender to "what is," and open ourselves to the inner lessons that then unfold.

Mindbody work gives you a key to unlock the door leading to the deep knowing of your potentials, which can then open many new and creative possibilities for expressing your true self. It is hard work. It is hard because you are so accustomed to fighting your way through problems that you feel are obstructing your progress. If someone disagrees with your opinion, for example, you may feel compelled to "argue to win." Dropping the fight means to allow room for all opinions to equally co-exist, which reduces stress dramatically. In effect, you take the pressure off yourself when you no longer need to win. It is difficult—almost beyond imagining—to lay down your weapons and let yourself experience the pain resulting from the tension itself. But it is essential to go into that experience. Until you do, the tension *cannot* be dissolved. By definition, if you are rigged up and ready to fight, the tension has its harbor, its reason for existence, and it perpetuates the constriction that you want to release.

GOING BEYOND THE STORY

It is important with emotions, as with a storyline in general, that you do not get too caught up in trying to define or "figure out" what emotion you are having. The challenge is to move away from categorical thinking. Naming emotions can sometimes give us a handle for conversation, and that is useful. It is convenient for us to say, "I feel anger" or "I feel sad" or "I feel fearful" when we are conversing with each other. But what really matters is to acknowledge the *sensations* associated with the emotion you are experiencing.

Certain sensations are associated with the constriction of energy moving through you, and the different nuances of that constriction are what we label emotion. The more you become accustomed to identifying the sensations you are feeling in the body, the more capable you will be to articulate your experience. However, working within the old therapy paradigm, we may think that by naming it we have cured it, and that is not the case. Fixing things outside yourself will not solve the problem, either. Sometimes circumstances do need to change, but that is beside the point here.

What we really need to do with the whole issue of emotions is to adopt an entirely new paradigm. We have grown accustomed to thinking of emotions as discrete entities that can be described and named. Instead, we might view emotions as energic patterns that reflect certain mental constructs. These mental constructs become our stories about how the world is and how we are within the world. In your search for wholeness, it is important not to seek to change the story and thus change the construct, but to move beyond the story and the construct entirely. The invitation is to recognize and not give energy to the conceptual framework that defines your inner—and therefore your outer—limits.

It is common wisdom that in any given experience every person in a room will usually tell a different story about what occurred. We make up stories to explain our internal experience. But if you define your future based on such a story, you are stuck in a cycle. Having made up a story, it becomes your self-definition or the definition of "how things are," and you become trapped in a repetition of that story. If you define your reality by your stories, by your history, you are not giving yourself any options. You cannot experience anything in your life other than what you have already experienced until you *allow something new into your life*. Remember that *you* are the creator of your stories, and your stories do not reflect ultimate reality. The stories you tell yourself and others are invitations to that which you allow into your life.

The path is to rest deeply inside the sensation you are having and not run away from it. Do not explain it away or blame it on anyone else. Go deeply into the sensation and acknowledge the constriction. Let the story with which you have explained your life to yourself dissolve. Let it become more fluid. Like magic, the emotion you think you are experiencing will transform. That is because the emotion you are experiencing is just a sensation in the body reflecting a particular fixed energy pattern. Emotion is energy moving against the barrier of the mental construct you have created and are living out as your reality.

Susan was 58 years old when she came to see me. She walked with a cane because her leg had been shattered in a car accident at age 20. She had been diagnosed with multiple sclerosis at age 39 after suffering symptoms of the disease for 20 years. She had seen numerous doctors over the years, but none had the complete picture of her symptoms because she was telling herself the story that they would write her off as a hypochondriac. By the time I saw her, she was suffering from acute back pain, migraine headaches, and trauma-induced osteoarthritis. She was also suffering from side-effects from the many drugs she was taking for her diverse symptoms, and she was severely depressed. She could not sleep because of the pain. Her inner critic was running her life and she felt useless. She saw herself as a victim of tragic circumstances—a story that was reflected in the life choices she made.

As we began our work together, Susan began to see where her story was running her life. Reflecting, through interactive imagery and gestalt therapy, she began to learn that there were things she could do to help herself—that she did not have to be the victim of her many physical symptoms. Instead of being stuck in the story of "I can't do anything anymore," she rediscovered how much she loved painting. She has not had a miraculous "cure," but now she sleeps better and has learned to live with her pain in a new way. She has also learned techniques to minimize the pain. Using imagery, meditation and acupressure, she is able to make a dramatic difference in her pain level. Most importantly, she recognizes her struggle as a spiritual journey and has a more positive outlook.

In attempting to disengage from a story you have told yourself, you may encounter several obstacles. The first obstacle is the dishonesty you have engaged in to maintain the storyline. I call it dishonesty only because it is a fabrication—it is not a blatant lie, but it is selective sight. Everything you see and experience goes through a conceptual framework. The fabric of your life becomes dense with the stories that exist in your mind, and you fear that letting go of any particular thread of that fabric will unravel your life.

It is terribly threatening to the storyline when you deselect or reselect or unselect elements in your stories, or even recognize the selectivity as an option. It can be unnerving to recognize that every person who plays a particular role in your life no longer holds a clear position in your mind, which means your relationship with that person is suddenly undefined. Additionally, when the script changes, it can be disorienting for everyone involved. For instance, if your husband is playing the part of the reactive bully who speaks harshly to your whining victim, and you no longer accept the role of victim, he can no longer play that part in your life.

The second obstacle you might face is the anxiety that occurs when you try to let go of your illusions about how you know *yourself* to be, as contained within the story. That anxiety can be nearly unbearable. Why? Because you know and accept yourself to be the role you are playing in the stories you are telling—it is that simple.

The myth has become your identity. Letting go of the story, then, requires a change in how you identify yourself.

Another difficulty in dropping the story is that certain individuals may have come into your life because they fit into the roles you need them to fulfill. You may have grown familiar with those who inhabit your life, and even if they play a negative role in your story, you may experience a horrible fear of loss. That is natural when you are faced with the discomforting potential of having people move out of your life. Women who are caught in abusive relationships, for example, often have that terrible sense of loss when they drop the victim storyline.

Finally, if you change your role in a story it means that, like Susan, you will have to accept more responsibility for your life. So wherever you have relegated yourself and your function to a familiar script, you will have to pause in the moment and allow a fresh perspective to emerge. This is at once liberating and frightening in its enormity. You must be more awake and fluid in the moment and recognize that you always have the ultimate choice about how to respond to a given situation. The solidity of the familiar is comforting, so breaking out of the pattern can be scary. For example, you can no longer relinquish responsibility to the familiar other who defines your reality for you because "that's the way I am." You must be willing to accept the discomfort of loss and let go of the fear associated with being responsible for yourself and your own life. You must be willing to live in the uneasiness that arises in the process of becoming disillusioned about who you are moment to moment. The Appendix offers some supportive techniques that will help you dare to be brave when encountering those elements of discomfort, resting with them until the transition happens.

Several qualities are extremely helpful to facilitate a shift in how you relate to your stories, and the first is a sense of trust in a bigger picture. Every religion and spiritual discipline talks about the need for death or dying in order to find ourselves. The process of disillusionment *is* a sensation of dying, and you cannot go there if you do not trust. Some might call that faith in a Higher Being. However you think about it, there needs to be some space into which you dare to surrender yourself as you know yourself to be. Then you can be reworked, reformatted, and freed from the painful constrictions and the lies you have told yourself.

That kind of faith requires tremendous courage, because it is the unknown into which you surrender. This is another layer of courage beyond what it takes, for instance, to move to a new town or begin a new career. The sort of courage I'm talking about is the courage it takes to surrender into the space where you do not know who you will be and you do not know who anybody else will be. You will be entering a space where you have not defined anything—it is like leaping off a cliff.

MORE ABOUT FACING THE FEAR

As mentioned, when you finally set aside your defenses and just breathe quietly, what often comes up is fear. You fear what will happen if you do not defend yourself. After all, if you do not fight, who will protect you? If you set down your weapons, your self-defeating behaviors, your fight language, your self-righteous behaviors, your justifications—if you set all that down, what are you left with? You are left with the terror, the sensation that you are not going to make it. Sitting with that sensation of terror takes the most tremendous courage imaginable. It will take however long it takes for the fear to pass, and there is no guarantee that you will immediately start feeling better. Of course you want to do all this because you want to feel better, so the fact that you have to sit through agony to get there is not particularly appealing! However, most spiritual traditions recognize that at some point the biggest barrier of all is the effort we make. Letting go of effort does not mean we sit passively in an attitude of helplessness—that is still fight energy turned inward, and it is still a barrier because it creates tension.

Fear exists in layers. The most obvious fear is the jitters, the anxiety you experience when you stop fighting and all the superficial reasons why you must go on fighting arise. That is just the outer layer, but you have to go through that to get to the deeper layers of fear. One of the deeper layers is our self-image—what we believe we really are—and we all have many aspects to that self-image. In the metaphor of the Garden of Eden, when Adam and Eve ate the apple, what they got was illusory thinking. As human beings, we define ourselves in relationship to every experience or person we encounter in our world. In every interaction, we carry with us an image of who we are relative to that situation or person. You must strip all that away. In letting go of your illusions about who you think you are relative to the world, relative to other people, relative to anything you think you want, you drop barriers to your authentic expression. Because these barriers define yourself to yourself, dropping them will produce fear at first.

If you drop the fight, you are stripped of your illusions. You fear being exposed for…what? *That* is what you must discover! Often at the center of all the layers of fear is a kernel of deep belief that is the most poignant and the most fearful. You will go through enormous shenanigans to avoid looking at it. Think about the distractions you use to avoid facing your illusions—television, noise, busyness, caffeine, sugar, alcohol, relationships, mall shopping. It does not matter what it is, anything that keeps you occupied and preoccupied is a distraction. When you drop the distraction and sink deeper, you will start to encounter, engage with, and expose the layers of fear about who you are, and who you might be, and what you might not be able to do, what you might represent, and so on and so forth. Expose them for what they are. They are just fears, but they are running your life. You will find that the kernel of fear in the middle of it all is some variation of "I'm bad" or "I'm not okay" or "There is something wrong with me" or "I can't." You will tap into some self negation that is so primordial and so basic that it is the original sin. That is where it all began. That is what kicked you out of the garden. That is why you cannot believe in yourself and why you cannot succeed in the ways you want to succeed.

These layers of fear, covered over by the images you have created out of that initial scar in your energy matrix, are what create the complexity in your life. You try to protect yourself in many ways—

staying overly busy, always being angry or rejecting, trying to make yourself acceptable by projecting the "nice guy" image, the "good girl" image, or the "highly successful" image. These are usually masks you present to the world, under which you try to hide your fear. So it is no mystery why good girls get headaches by the end of the day and good boys get heart attacks. When you exist for any length of time within the constraints of such internal dialogue and tension, no matter how well hidden, it inevitably takes its toll on the body. The masks you use to "be acceptable" in the face of that which you deny only complicates the matter because sooner or later the body truly will reflect in tangible form the internal dynamics you habitually play out. Hiding the facets of yourself you do not like behind a façade not only does not solve the problem, it makes it worse by keeping you from accessing the deeper level where you can make a difference—and heal.

The hard work comes from experiencing the sensations that arise as you thaw out the frozen complexities. It is excruciatingly painful. In our culture we have grown accustomed to anesthetizing ourselves, to relieving our pain. We want more relief, more distractions, so we add more and more layers. The human mind is uniquely equipped to live in fantasy—the stories we make up as explanations for our situation. Within the framework of these stories, we tend to frame ourselves in complimentary ways that keep us out of the muck of facing our inner tensions.

Mindbody work requires the opposite approach, and not many people want to do it. Because the body carries the full repertoire of our internal states without the benefit of the lies our minds convince us of, reentering the full, naked awareness of our organic selves can be quite a shock. Most people are forced into it by a crisis where they are ripped open. The shell can shatter in various ways when we are forced to see with some degree of awareness those parts of ourselves we do not want to face. For example, we can be shorn of our self-image by the loss of a job, a mate, or a life situation. Sometimes these losses take us deeper into that core of our self.

When we are forced to look down into our core and find ourselves empty of all the images we had of ourselves, we often find it difficult to retain that new awareness. We tend to rebuild life around the familiar again. So we hear people say things like, "We were so bonded as a community after the hurricane went through…after I lost my house… after I discovered I had cancer." But life continues, and we go back to the familiar patterns we know. That is where we find the challenge and complexity in mindbody work—staying connected with what truly is, staying awake.

A NEW WAY OF BEING

Going beyond the story means to approach life with a sense of adventure. As you let go, you will develop curiosity and a sense of openness toward whatever life presents to you. You will redefine the pain and darkness as a feeling of potential instead of tensing up and fighting it. You will be able to gracefully let go and accept an unknown future.

You will be brave in greeting yourself as a new friend. When you have the courage to drop your story, you meet yourself again and again and you are okay with whoever you find yourself to be. If you let go, you are bound to see the next layer of self-definition. Be patient with yourself, because there are many layers, and it is a process. You are brave in welcoming the stranger—you greet the new you with an open heart. You dare to have an experience that is authentically different from anything that you have experienced before.

Sara, a client who saw me for assistance in dealing with irritable bowel syndrome, revealed this awareness beautifully. After a session in which she had done particularly deep work facing the intense constrictions she carried in her body related to her relationship with her father, she remarked on how she felt "like something major that seemed like part of me is missing." Sitting for a moment on the edge of the table, Sara reflected, "You know, the biggest challenge right now for me really is to not go looking for the familiar painful feeling again." It takes courage to dare to experience ourselves as fundamentally missing some aspect by which we have created an identity.

With this bravery comes a deeper humility and a heart-centered friendliness to all you meet. You choose love with whatever you find. You let go of the constriction that protects you from seeing whatever it was you did not want to see. This is the heart of the matter: above all else, to be committed to encountering everything in your life, including yourself, with loving kindness.

A BALANCING ACT

One of the underpinnings to a sense of wholeness, and therefore wellness, is balance. But let's look at what that really means. I frequently hear people say, "I wish I had a more balanced life"—as if it were a static sort of thing. Balance is not static. For example, you can stand on one foot and you might appear stable, but in actuality all the muscles in that foot are wiggling like crazy even as you rest in the awareness of being centered. Things are constantly changing. If you judge yourself negatively because you notice you are wiggling while standing on one foot, you will most likely tense up and topple over. The irony is that if you just accept the wiggling and make whatever adjustments are necessary, you can continue to stand that way indefinitely. To surrender into the notion of balance means to recognize that a corrective force is needed on a continual basis. In fact, just accepting the idea helps you come into balance much more quickly.

As another example, our human reaction to a strong emotion like grief is to want to get rid of it. But if you never allow yourself to fully experience grief, it will remain to fester inside you, begging through your unconscious awareness to be released, and you will never feel the open heart of joy. When you truly let yourself feel betrayal or the pain of loss, you wake up one day and find that you have been carried into a deeper awareness of yourself and that your heart has opened in a new way. However, you cannot know that sweetness if you have not allowed yourself to go to into the darkness. Conversely, if you wallow in or indulge the darkness, you will never come through to the light of joy. To cling to the state of feeling blue is just as dysfunctional as to reject it outright. It is a balancing act of accepting "what is" to be as it is, while remaining open to change.

When you recognize the dynamic nature of all your sensations and emotions, you can fully be with them and allow them to gracefully pass on when they have done their transformative work on you. You are not attached to the form of the emotion or circumstance, but instead recognize it as yet one more face of the ever-changing flow of life.

The Chinese yin yang symbol (*Figure 1*) wonderfully represents this idea of balance. Neither the feminine aspect of yin (darkness, wetness, coldness) nor the masculine aspect of yang (activity, lightness, dryness) are static states. Yin and yang define one another. One can only be defined *in relationship to* the other. This is a subtle but profound concept. As the symbol teaches, at the point where either yin or yang is at its strongest, it automatically contains and becomes the other.

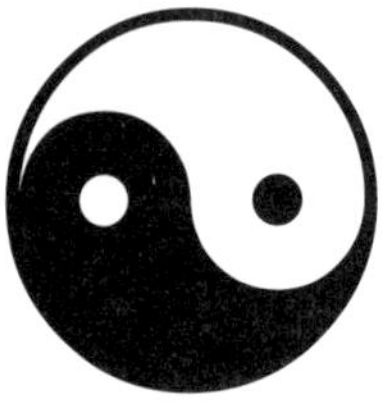

Figure 1

For convenience, throughout this book I will talk about the individual aspects of our wholeness—physical health, mental wellbeing, emotional wellness, relational balance, and a sense of purpose. Remember that these aspects are contained within the totality of who we are and they are not ultimately separate. Just like in the yin yang symbol, the state of one aspect defines the other aspect. If we are out of balance in one area, by definition that means we are out of balance in another area. Finding our true center requires constant "wiggling" to remain whole and healthy.

Life is constantly changing. In finding balance, you will sometimes look a little messy and ungraceful. Once you accept the truth of that idea, you will receive the power, energy, and strength to do what you need to do to come back to balance. You make the necessary changes from within the effortless state of surrender into the Tao, into *Shen*, into the path, into the will of God.

CHAPTER 3

Mental Constructs: the blocks to wellness

As mentioned in the last chapter, the tension you carry in your body is a physical manifestation of the mental constructs you have absorbed and memorized in your neural network. You are a complete "package deal" of energic complexes. These complexes comprise a physical component in addition to an emotional component and you experience this matrix as your identity. When you are at your best, these energic complexes are reflected in a dynamic and fluid way, but when you have memorized a fixed pattern as part of your identity, you are trapped. You must wake up to these patterns in order to free yourself from them.

Most of us identify with various complexes that include the physical structure but are not limited to it. It might involve a function or position in life, a circumstance, environment, or relationships to people and things. These components of your identity can be ultimately destroyed if threatened, so every single point of identification you have is a possible place of fear where you harbor tension, guardedness, and a learned response. The more you are identified with any given "thing" and the more intense the relationship, the harder it is to let go.

As things move and shift and change inside yourself, you will lose your sense of identity in relationship to the outside world. To the extent you have identified yourself with anything as a solid substance or a fact, you lose fluidity. Either you are clinging to it ("Ah, this is me, you can't take it away!") or you want to hide it ("Oh, this is me, I don't want them to see this!"). You make yourself a noun, and you are not. You are a verb. You are the act of life living itself. That which can be identified as a separate "you" is simply a point of awareness. If you think you are a solid state, look at your baby picture and compare that to what you see when you look in the mirror! What part of you is solid?

As humans, we seem to have a terrific need to describe ourselves in a way that is identifiable. We want a point of reference to call our self. We think we need to matter to others as a separate entity. However, that sense of separateness is precisely what causes our misery. It cannot last, and it will not last. Most spiritual teachers say that someday you must die to your life as you know it and be born again into a new life. It is not life that ends, it is your sense of separateness. You must die to that sense of separation, and the way to get there is to confront, embrace, and allow the dissolution of every mental construct you have embodied. What a joy that is, when you have truly surrendered!

RECOGNIZING YOUR MENTAL CONSTRUCTS

How do you know what your mental constructs are? You notice the sensations in your body. You find your points of anxiety. You breathe into the anxiety and describe it in terms of the tension you hold in your body. You breathe into the tension and allow your breath to carry you deeper until you get into the inner membrane of fear that is the descriptor of who you think you are—that identity you are trying to protect or to defend yourself against. And then you rest in that place of misery until the breath in and the breath out begin to dissolve the self and you become aware that it is only an image. It is a powerful image, because it has defined the construct of your life, but it is not any more solid than what you make it out to be.

Let's use the state of anxiety as an example of how this works. Take a moment to recall a situation where you felt anxious. Pay attention to what happens in your body as you recall the experience. Notice the sensations that are associated with it. Although the experience may vary slightly in different people, you will likely notice very specific sensations. You may notice tension around the diaphragm, in your upper back, your hands, or your jaws. It will probably be a feeling of "holding on for dear life." These patterns of tension lie on the "fault line" of the underlying mental construct. In other words, every mental-emotional pattern has a corresponding "usual" physical manifestation or way of expressing in the body.

As you stay with that sense of tension, you will begin to notice certain reactive stances, and an emotion will undoubtedly arise. For example, if you are holding tension in your diaphragm and your middle back, you will sense a barrier to the free flow of breath and you may feel angry. If you go more deeply into the awareness, you will discover the beliefs that obligate the body to hold itself in that particular pattern. Going deeper still, you will discover the idea of being in danger. The reaction might be, "I need to be prepared to fight." Somebody or something is threatening to you and you do not feel safe. Something is about to be shattered or scattered and you feel obligated to defend yourself. As you break through the barriers of tension that are reflected as outer anxiety, the core belief system—the inner membrane to the mental construct—begins to arise, and you discover fear as your predominant state of being. Fear typically revolves around a sense that the self is about to be destroyed, and the learned behavior is a protective device. In this case, the protective device is the angry, defensive posture. If you continue going deeper into this construct, via the fear, eventually you will discover a sense of emptiness, a sense of questioning, a sense of not knowing who you are. The fear of surrendering into that space of emptiness is so overwhelming that most people will go to great lengths to avoid entering it. But is it precisely this final surrender that leads us to the knowing of who we really are—the Space, the Peace, the Love from which *all* form has originated.

Besides anger, another fear response might be to avoid or run away. The anxiety might express itself as a feeling of panic and increased energy along the spine, or a sense of jitteriness. Let yourself rest in that state of anxiety long enough to be delivered into the inner membrane of fear within it. Rest long enough to sink down more deeply and feel it in the body. You may feel as if ants were crawling inside your body, making it so you can hardly stand to be in your own skin. You will want to be anywhere but where you are. To avoid it, you may want to distract yourself, chatter, go do this or that, rather than experience the sensation of your cells jumping around as they do in this predicament. Stay with it, breathe, allow yourself to focus, and recognize that whatever you are experiencing is a passing phenomenon. It comes and goes. Notice the rapid arising and falling in waves. Allow yourself to sink deeper and you may notice a sensation in the lower part of your back, your pelvis, or your lower abdomen—somewhere in the first chakra. Stay there; stay with it. Sooner or later, the pains you are trying to avoid with this kind of anxiety—the deep nest of pain, beliefs, and programming that you have accepted as your basic identity—will begin to come to the surface.

Your defense may also show up in a desire to hide. Much chronic pain that exists in the world is the result of being stuck in this desire. It is born out of trying to prove to yourself and to the world that you are not what you believe yourself to be. That push and pull creates a horrible state of chronic pain. Chronic low back pain in particular often reflects this predicament. Sooner or later, as you rest in the belief of your unacceptability, the tension and the intensity will begin to lessen. First it comes in bits, then in a more encompassing awareness. You will manage to get a breath, a space of fresh air, a realization. You will understand that this is not who you are—it is an image, a belief. It is a mental construct that is wrapped around you with its tentacles tightly holding you in the pattern you call your life. Because it is so abhorrent, you have been protecting yourself from seeing it and trying to hide it from others. You have forced yourself to accept layer upon layer upon layer of lies in order to protect yourself.

This brief, rather simplistic description belies the difficulty of actually entering into and walking through this level of surrender. Recognizing the false self can take years, and most people avoid it for a lifetime, because the demise of the ego that is required to enter into the void is horrifying. After all, if you give up your identity, it means completely not knowing who you are for a while. That is terrifying, and most people find it completely unacceptable. The sensation is sometimes described as a fear of death, but it is actually worse than physical death. It is not the fear of losing your physical structure that is so scary—unless you are so identified with your physical structure that it is all you know yourself to be—it is fear of the unknown, of nonexistence. It takes great courage and deep faith to face this fear, but once you have begun to move through the different points of identification, the relief that comes with being in that state of emptiness is sweet indeed. You begin to embrace the emptiness as deep potential, and it all becomes much easier.

GIVING UP THE FIGHT

Pushing against or resisting anything ensures its continuance. This is an ancient recognition from Buddhist thought that is proven by a basic physics principles—anything you push against will push back with precisely equal energy. So if you want something to disappear, quit fighting! It is that simple. If you do not resist it, it will dissolve and you will discover it is not there.

You are so used to fighting the horrible dragons that you think are out to get you, but all the while the dragons are contained in the fabric of your being through the mental constructs you have created. Of course, you will be able to find "proof" that the dragons are real and exist outside yourself. If you have a fight to pick, you will find somebody who will fight with you. If there are fifty people in a room and one person is emanating the source of energy that would buy in to exactly the fight you need, you will gravitate to that person.

It is a magnetic pull. It matches your energy in quantity, quality, and frequency. We are all energy bodies and the energy patterns predictably play themselves out, finding a perfect match. There is a certain perfection in this, so do not fight the circumstances you are in. Embrace whatever you encounter. Ultimately, you could say you brought yourself there by the magnetic pull of whatever it is inside you that is longing to wake up. So fight your battles carefully, recognizing that what you are really fighting is your own sense of self.

If there is something you long to be and you doubt your potential to express it, you will surely find someone who will bring those doubts to the surface. You will find yourself in a fight, trying to prove hard that which you want everybody to know is true about you. You will be given the opportunity to vent this vehemently as much as you need to until you just accept it.

If you are terribly afraid that something is true about you and you do not want it to be true, such as the messages you got from your parents when you were younger, you will almost certainly be in a defensive posture, trying to disprove that "truth." The beauty is that as you awaken, you no longer need to project these arguments onto other people. You just pay attention to the voices in your head and recognize them as the illusory concepts they are.

SHAME AND BLAME

Unfortunately, the intention to do harm is contained within each of us. Most of us will deny it with our last breath, but it is there. We all hate some aspect of ourselves, and thus the intention to do harm is directed against the self and is reflected as shame. On the outside, you carry around your protective defenses to prove to the world that whatever it is you are ashamed of, your personal secret, really is not there. But underneath that protective layer, the shame—a direct aggression against the self—exists. Spiritual practices and psychological tools abound to eradicate the shame about whatever it is you find unacceptable about yourself. Instead, it is far better to embrace it, to sit with the shame and bring to it the energy of loving kindness.

Loving kindness, compassion, and acceptance comprise the antidote to it all. And that which you are most ashamed of, you most need to accept. That does not mean you accept it as the reality of who you are, because you will discover it is not who you are. But you cannot come to that awareness without accepting the unacceptable first.

Here we are back in the world of paradox. When you deeply and completely and fully accept whatever it is that you are most dreading and most ashamed of, it will change into something else. However, this gets tricky, because you cannot get there by trying to change it. You cannot fool yourself by trying to accept it in order to make it change! You must truly embrace it with the deep, completely compassionate heart of the *bodhisattva*[4]. And then it transforms, because it is not really there. It is your imagination fighting with itself.

If that unacceptable part of yourself is so horrifying you dare not even look at it, if you cannot even bear the suspicion that you contain that within yourself, you will direct the hatred, the animosity, and the intent to do harm outside yourself. That is called blame. You find a target against which you can cast your harmful energy, your anger, your name calling, or your aversion. The psychological term for this is projection. You project onto someone or something else your deepest fear of what you might be. Your mental constructs can be part of a family or community issue and a shared story, and that shared story becomes the community dynamics, the national borders and identities, the arguments, and the wars. But your actual work begins inside. It all begins with that which you deem acceptable or unacceptable. The whole storyline gets carried forward and becomes the myths you pass on to your children, who then carry that energy pattern—the family story—forward into the next generation. We have family stories and we have national stories, and each of our stories contains the energy patterns in a full-blown, dramatized, and entertaining fashion. These patterns are so familiar and predictable that we make plays and movies and television shows out of them and most people laugh at the same place and feel tense at the same place.

WORKING WITH COMPLEXES

Working with your mental complexes is the foundational process through which you will gain your freedom. A simple mantra you can use to remember how to work with these constructs is: *face, embrace, and allow space.* In other words, when you become aware of any tension, anger, anxiety, or other ripple that interferes with your harmonious interrelationship with life, face it. Notice it and squarely face it. If you entertain the possibility of running away from, fighting, overcoming, or in any way resisting that which is difficult for you, you create tension. That tension becomes an energetic barrier around the phenomenon, which increasingly intensifies and solidifies the construct. You literally create an energetic entity out of those facets of pain you resist, and that entity becomes the enemy.

Science has recently shown that if a researcher encloses a body of molecules in a container, after some varying amount of time the molecules will coalesce into some sort of form, creating a dynamic entity. We see a similar phenomenon in mega structures like corporations, bureaucracies, and so forth. If you have ever had difficulty trying to intelligently engage with such an entity to get a simple answer or to change something, you will recognize the challenge you are facing. This kind of difficulty occurs because the entity allows very little freedom for a given individual to think or act independently. You will see this phenomenon happening on all levels within the entity of your self. You are an aggregate of molecules spinning around some notion of self, and the entities of negativity are created in a similar fashion. Every facet of yourself that you resist and create energy around develops a sense of form that feeds on negativity. The old-fashioned spiritual notion of "devil" is rooted in the awareness that it is as if something outside you takes over. It feels that way because it truly is not you, it is the negative energy that has taken form. In physics, the negative is the magnetic polarity that pulls to itself that which forms around it. Your resistance creates a form with structure and cohesiveness, and its "magnetic pull" can take you over.

An example of how this works might be when you have picked a fight and later you cannot understand why in heaven's name you said what you said. It is because the "entity" was having its way with you. It has a life of its own and was trying to get nourishment from yet another battle. Once the pattern has developed, it is very difficult to eradicate because inherent within it is a sense of continuity and trajectory—and a fear of loss. You fear the loss of control because you have identified yourself with these long-standing patterns and you feel as if you will lose yourself if you let go of them. But when Jesus said you must die to find yourself, he meant it. You must die to every single facet of yourself with which you are identified.

After squarely facing the construct, you must embrace it. In direct contrast to therapy as it has been practiced for the last few decades, do not attempt to overthrow, do not attempt to talk yourself out of anything, do not attempt to change your mind, do not attempt to do anything with these structures you have created. What you must do instead is to embrace the phenomenon. It has been said that what you resist persists. You allow yourself to be free of it by not resisting. Open your heart and take into yourself that which you most fear, just as you would lovingly encircle a beloved child who is hurting. You must do the same for any enemies you have created, because they merely represent what you have denied in yourself. If you deny anything in yourself, it is a given that you will project it onto someone else.

Finally, allow some space around the construct. Locate the tension in your body. Allow a gentle curiosity to develop. Ask "What is this? I genuinely want to know." Given this space, this lack of resistance, the construct will change. It has to, because it was your creation to begin with. It may take time, and these reactive patterns may recur, but the dynamic will simplify over time. In fact, the dynamic itself will begin to embrace you, and you will feel your self begin to dissolve. You will be taken over by the Life Force, which is eager to dissolve resistance to Itself. If you invite It in, It is there for you. As Jesus said, "Ask and it will be given to you; seek and you will find; knock and the door shall be opened to you."

Do not expect to find the answer all in a blinding flash or look for the challenge to suddenly disappear. Instead, life will gradually become simpler over time. You will probably continue to come up against the construct. But as long as you are practicing this type of surrender, a reaction does not necessarily mean you are regressing. You may be meeting the next layer of fear.

Be aware that you contain within yourself the archetypal history of the entire race, gender, and culture into which you were born. Consequently, the phenomena you experience in your body may not directly correlate with your lifetime or your actions. You may contain tensions and reactive patterns that do not make any sense to you at all. Do not try to make sense of them—that is never the point of the practice. Simply face, embrace, and allow space. In this way, you are healing the human culture itself. Likewise, as you work through those personal issues you can readily identify, you will eventually enter them at a deeper level and begin to heal at the level of race, gender, and culture. Your life will take on an archetypal meaning and then you are truly a healer of the human race.

It is not that the pain necessarily goes away; it just becomes easier because you recognize the pattern and you surrender more readily. You no longer take anything personally. You will become gentle with yourself as you find life happening *through* you, not *to* you. Compassion begins to vibrate in every cell of your body. People may comment on it. They may say that when you walk in, peace comes with you. Do not take this personally, either. You will eventually get to the point where you no longer experience yourself as a separate entity. You will still have a body. You still fall asleep, wake up, and do your day, but everything is quite changed. Your experience of life is very different.

THE LARGER PICTURE

For a long time, an argument has existed about whether humans are the product of nature or nurture. It is both and neither. Each of us is a unique point of awareness born into a particular set of circumstances and we carry a particular energy pattern in our DNA. The energy dynamics are encoded within a whole energy matrix into which we come. That is why astrology can be accurate if done correctly—it is simply a description of energy patterns. It is not cause and effect; it is not the alignment of the stars that creates a particular situation. Instead, certain energy dynamics are being played out on the planet at any given time and the human beings that are born at that time perfectly reflect those dynamics through our design. Our design *is* that energy pattern being played out on the earth's plane such that each of us will encounter in physical form that which will help us to wake up.

To some extent, we need this externalization in order to wake up. Energy patterns interacting with themselves do not get very far without some anchor, and our bodies are that anchor. Our bodies are the path, and our circumstances are no mistake. We must shed the constrictions that have changed the free flow of energy into painful constructs that turn life against itself in dreadfully painful ways. The whole point is to free up the life energy and return to the awareness of ultimate peace. We are all trying to wake up to that remembrance.

When you are enlightened, it is not that you disappear in a ball of light—it is that light resonates through every cell of your body. Your DNA is vibrating with the sheer joy of life, and you experience pain differently. You recognize it joyfully as that next edge inviting life to move through you as a conduit for healing the human race. You give yourself over to that completely because that is why you are here. If you are reading this and you are resonating with it, you can count on it. This is why you are here, so surrender. Let it go. Face, embrace, allow space.

You are the portal. You are the doorway. You are the threshold. You are the action. You are the path. You are life experiencing Itself. You are Life returning to Itself. You are life itself.

CHAPTER 4

Relationships: the field of play

*R*elationship is a mental construct. When you have completely surrendered and know that Life is One, relationship changes its meaning entirely. However, it is impossible to believe you are a separate being and not be in relationship with everything else as seemingly separate entities. You experience yourself in relationship constantly, with every breath you breathe. Right now, you are in relationship with this book, and the book is in relationship with you—it is always a two-way street. When you realize that fundamental truth, you begin to open yourself to the possibility of the moment. You allow life to present itself to you in its fullest form, moment to moment.

You are magnetically attracted to exactly those persons and circumstances that will most effectively activate your core issues. When you experience conflict with another person, it is because you are projecting the cause of your upset onto them. When you fail to recognize the origin of suffering as a mental construct you do not want to own, it becomes like a shadow that is cast on those around you. When you look at those individuals through this perceptual filter—this shadow—it appears as if it is *they* who have "the problem."

You are capable of recognizing only that which you perceive through the filter of your belief system, and that perceptual filter is framed within the context of your mental constructs. In other words, you hear what you believe, you see what you believe, and you feel what you believe. "Reality" as defined by these limits varies from person to person. Paying attention to the dynamics in relationships can be a gateway into the belief structures that hold you captive, because relationships activate the reactive spaces that are the clue to your shadow. These reactive tendencies tell you the truth about where you need to search for your mental constructs. Romantic relationships have the greatest magnetic pull and so they most deeply activate these reactive tendencies. However, the same thing occurs at some level in all relationships.

A DANCE OF POLARITIES

Deep within you is an enormous well of loneliness spawned from the desire to merge in awareness with the Source of life. The desire for merging with another human being reflects this yearning. Conversely, you contain the desire to be a unique, separate self (your ego self). In psychology, having a strong ego is recognized as a healthy thing, because only by being completely separate can you have the actuality of experience. But you are being called back home, to wholeness. You can actuate that wholeness to the extent you recognize what stands in the way of fully accepting all aspects of your being.

Usually, shortly after the initial glow of a new romantic relationship wears off, we are exposed to all the apparent differences, and we view them as "problems." These "problems" are simply thinly disguised shadow faces dancing for our attention and ultimate acceptance. Every time we choose to act from love in the face of conflict with our dearly beloved, we accept back into our awareness at a deeper level more of the fullness and essence of Life itself. We are returning home.

Everyone contains both "masculine" and "feminine" energies. When you identify yourself as male or female—as a role with certain dictates that deny the existence of the opposite in yourself—you erect barriers that keep you from fully actuating your potential or fully merging with your "opposite" as a couple. As a female, you must recognize and completely accept the masculine within you. As a male, you must recognize and completely accept your feminine aspects. For example, a male must accept his receptive aspects, and a female must accept her assertive tendencies. This is simplistic, but reflects the general dynamic. When you completely accept the polarities within yourself, the merging between male and female will nourish you rather than drain you. It is possible for the masculine and feminine to merge in a unique way so the energies reflect and enhance one another at the most fundamental level.

When you can fully accept what you find inside as well as outside yourself, you have dropped your ego, because your ego is simply the belief that you are separate. As you allow the shadow to be whatever it is, there are no longer any aspects of yourself or an apparent "other" to fight. You recognize, organically and in actuality, that we are One—not "as one," but truly One. The sensation of romantic love is a glimpse into this recognition of oneness. When you recognize the opposites *within* yourself, you will learn to dance within these polarities gracefully and peacefully in the world.

EMBRACING RELATIONSHIP CHALLENGES

Many theories exist about what goes into attraction. Some say the chemistry of pheromones induces a hormonal attraction. Some say you are attracted to someone who reminds you of your mother/father so that you can work through the unfinished business you have with them. These are not mutually exclusive statements. They are all part of who you are. You were born into a complex energy matrix, and your issues have been with you since birth, so of course the one who reminds you of your mother/father conglomerate is most likely to reflect those issues you contain within that matrix. It is important not to get too simplistic and think of this in terms of cause and effect, but you can learn a lot by looking at the patterns you had with your parents. These patterns reflect what is up for healing. You can also look at patterns in those with whom you are in committed relationships, such as your mate or best friend or business partners. But do not worry about clearing your issues with your parents or partners or friends—worry about clearing your issues within yourself.

It is also helpful to reflect on how love was defined and played out in your family of origin—not as a point of blame or an explanation for how you came into this predicament of yourself, but rather as a reflection your mental patterning. For example, people say things like "Love hurts." Well, that is never true—it is a belief about love that was developed because of certain past conditioning. So it is helpful to look at what beliefs you have about love that foster separation. Identify the errors in your thinking that need correction, and surrender deeply into the energies of a one-to-one relationship. If you can do that, it can help you in a very focused way.

The invitation to the deepest possibility of love is available in a primary committed relationship, and anything that causes separation between you and your partner is an impediment to love. *Anything* you do to avoid dealing with what is in front of you fosters a sense of separation, no matter how you frame it and what you call it. For example, you might say, "I need my own time and my own life." Is that true? Is it possible that you are running away from love? That is not to say that needing time out to get a handle on what is ailing you is not a good idea as a "time out" so you can catch your projections. But if the "time out" is actually avoidance of what is calling you into love's deepest embrace, you need to realize that. Individuation can be used as a form of running away from yourself. If you deeply accept every single facet of yourself, you will be able to accept it in another. But you can fool yourself and use that concept as a way of avoiding facing what is difficult. That is narcissism, and there is a difference. This is difficult to accept, because it is exactly what you do not want to see.

Whatever you do, do not view your issues as a "problem" or take them personally or let yourself go into shame because you have things to deal with. If you did not have issues, you would not be here! You are simply an energy form. You are a point of awareness. Your passage through time is, by definition, temporary. Of course, if you like solving problems and it helps to see it that way—like solving a crossword or putting together a puzzle—go for it. Think of it as your challenge, your task. Or you can think of it as your greatest gift to deal with in this lifetime. You might think, "Oh good, here's an issue. I've been looking for you, come on in!" Hold it in whatever way helps you get on with your healing. Be joyous in embracing and working through the issues that arise.

The ultimate purpose of any relationship is to surrender completely into the state of love. At the beginning of a romantic alliance, you resonate with this awareness. Everything in you is tuned in. Your soul has activated in you the awareness that you have the possibility of waking up to the fullness of love, merging back into life itself, and surrendering completely any sense of separation. We all long for that. But what happens then? In the magnificent force field of that powerful attraction, what is pulled out of you from your depths is everything that is in the way of that final merging. That is when the trouble begins—the challenges come, one after the other. The honeymoon is over, so to speak.

This is where you have the opportunity to recognize the blessing in your challenges. Now is the time to roll up your sleeves and get to work. First, you must quit blaming. Do not blame yourself, do not blame your parents, do not blame your partner, do not blame anybody. Once you are in the field of blame, everybody gets hit—it is like shrapnel. Instead, let it all go. As mentioned previously, blame and shame are the head and the tail of the same force, the same constriction. The challenge is the blessing, the invitation. This is actually a very simple rule, but it is profoundly difficult to put into practice, isn't it? If it were easy, you would not be in this predicament in the first place.

If you feel angry, or hear yourself accusing or ridiculing or wanting the other to be different, that is the clue that you are seeing some aspect of your own shadow. If you feel conflict, it is coming from within your own energy matrix. When you hear yourself making a judgment about another person, whether you are saying it out loud or just thinking it, stop. Say exactly the same thing about yourself. Do this internally, not necessarily to the other person. Accept that your judgment is about yourself. For example, if you say, "You never listen to me," stop and turn it around. (By the way, one clue that you are caught in your shadow is that you use words like "always" or "never.") Say instead, "I am not listening to me" or "I am not listening to you." This is your wake-up opportunity. What will surface is the thing you least want to see.

The clue to having hit a mental construct is that you will feel a "charge." That word is useful to remember, because it quite aptly describes what is going on. Your reaction will have some energy behind it, like a spark of electricity, and that reaction is probably a bit stronger than what most people outside your circumstance would think is warranted by the situation.

So what happens next? When a certain level of intimacy has been achieved and both individuals are committed to this process, you can have a conversation about what is happening. This works best when the couple has agreed that the relationship is a safe space in which to work through their issues together. The relationship allows space for these elements to come up, to be revealed, and to be owned. However, remember that protecting the space is not the same as protecting yourself from your own issues—in fact it is profoundly different. You must take responsibility, and never expect the other to take care of your issues for you. We often want our partner to take away our pain. But our partners cannot do for us what we will not do for ourselves.

"Co-dependency" is a psychological term that usually refers to a maladaptive method of coping with one another's demands and needs by dysfunctionally ignoring our own. This is in contrast to "interdependency," in which each person's needs are considered simultaneously and equally. Unfortunately, confusion about these two similar but profoundly different states can turn you away from the possibility of deep surrender. There is something not quite fulfilling when two people are insisting that they maintain themselves as separate, individually realized selves. When you do wholly surrender into love—which contains both you and your partner equally and safely—you will experience the merging you hunger for.

You were created male and female for a reason, and it was not just to procreate children.* Coupling is the form within which you can most deeply surrender into a merging that mimics the return home like nothing else on this three-dimensional plane can. It serves as a continually recurring invitation to surrender to love when fear or resistance arises. That is why romantic love and the sexual drive are so profoundly strong. It is the strongest element that exists. As such, it also has the strongest fear base. As discussed earlier, you fear-extinction, the loss of self. It is a fear based in reality, because that is exactly what will happen when you completely surrender. Your sense of an individual, separate self *will* disappear.

Paradoxically, you cannot experience complete fulfillment as long as you maintain a sense of separate self, but the sense of separate self is essential in order to begin the process of accepting all that is contained within you. When you accept every facet of yourself without apology, without shame, and without needing to blame the other, you—who you believe yourself to be—"disappears." The fear is natural—it is the protection you create around yourself to keep from losing who you think you are. The invitation into the full merging of a couple brings up that very fear.

You have forgotten who is in charge of the kingdom. Remember, *Shen* is the ruler of the kingdom, and *Shen* rests in your heart. The pull from your heart, the desire for merging heart-to-heart, will bring you back home. Once you have surrendered completely, your heart opens and there is no facet of life from which you are separate again. You are in love with life, and life is in love with you. Out of recognizing and accepting the polarities, your love for all beings is complete. Romantic love is that first intimation of the light and the bliss of which you are capable. The path back to that light and bliss can be long, winding, and difficult, but the more you can own your own issues without shame or apology, the faster you will get there.

So be glad when your partner pushes your buttons! Those are the "on" buttons—the electrical switches. When the charge is high, that

---

* The male/female polarities exist in both men and women in different ways, so some in same gender pairings are fulfilling these same principles.

is the fire energy welcoming you into the possibility of burning up all that stands in the way of your healing. It is painful, but that is only because you are frozen.

What you think you want more than anything is to be loved and appreciated for who you think you are. But you are mistaken about who you are! You are not your identity. If you want a list of who you are not, start with your name, then list every single function you perform in life. None of it is who you are. Anything that has the capacity to be threatened is not who you are. The love relationship is so powerful because as a person gets closer to you they will perhaps argue with your sense of identity. Recognize the gift in that. Who you are cannot be threatened by anyone's opinion, attitude, or conjecture. Who you truly are is infinite life. So when you feel threatened, recognize the tension, the barrier, and give silent gratitude. Embrace the charge that has you poised to fight back. Take a deep breath and allow the fury of that fire to penetrate right into that which you are not and burn it out. Focus on gratitude and allow space. Instead of using the fire in defense of what is not true, use it for the dissolution of what is not true.

There will come a time when you are able to use the energy contained within each emotion for its pure purpose. Anger energy, for example, is the fire that tells the truth unwaveringly and clearly. To learn how to use it safely in the outside world, you must first apply it to yourself, which means your anger is never in self-defense. If you use anger in self-defense, you have misapplied it. Anger energy is clear and concise. It tells the truth without apology and without fear.

RESPONSIBILITY

Being responsible in a spiritual context should not be viewed as being obligated. Having an obligation is like having a huge weight around your neck. Unfortunately, religions build on this sense of responsibility. You can let go of that interpretation of being responsible. Perhaps a better way to think of it is being accountable—keeping agreements. In this sense, responsibility holds you to the fire of your own transformation.

You are responsible for feeling fully, embracing completely, and seeking the truth at all times. You might think of living with a sense of responsibility as work, but it is a different definition of work. It seems like work because it keeps you right on your growing edge, keeping you answerable for your own arguments, your own barricades. Being responsible is remaining truthful in every moment, moment to moment.

In the Chinese meridian system, responsibility is reflected in the liver/gall bladder meridian, which feeds into *Shen*, the heart. Responsibility transforms you and deposits you right into the fullness of your true being, which is *Shen*. This kind of responsibility reflects complete surrender and allows the emperor of the kingdom—not your ego self—to be in charge. The kingdom—the field of play—is your relationships. It is Tao, the dance of life.

WHEN THE HONEYMOON ENDS

Although it happens in the context of relationship, the awakening process is an individual journey, which means that each person in the relationship can do only their own internal work. Because of the delicious nectar in the beginning of a romantic relationship, you might wish you could, or think you can, stay there forever. But there may come a time when there is a lack of resonance such that the issues are no longer aptly activated for one or the other partner. Relationship is always co-created, so as issues resolve, there is mutuality in the shift that occurs. Forms may come and go, but there is always perfection in the dance.

On the other hand, what often happens is that at the first blush of difficulty, you think love has disappeared. Love is never absent. Love is what keeps your heart beating. Love is who you are. Recognize that first blush for what it is—the initiation phase—and be willing to let that go when the time comes. Be happy when the challenges begin to surface because that is an indication you have moved into the next phase of your own evolution. Embrace it with a sense of joy. Anticipate it. Reframe the whole romantic experience so you can willingly move forward together. When you freak out and think, "Oh, we need counseling, we need divorce," that may be true. But do not misidentify the challenges as they come up as necessarily the end of your romance. The chemistry and energetic bonding that occurs in the initial phase is crucial, but do not frantically try to prolong it with wine and supper and music. Yes, nourish the joy of your relationship, just do not misidentify those early syrupy feelings as all there is.

As you work through your issues together, you will experience a much deeper state of merging and love like nothing you can imagine. You will experience a complete trust and surrender, and the joy of being completely known for who you really are. You will see yourself reflected in your partner's eyes. This is the essence of "needing" a partner to do this work.

SURRENDER

Whatever you find as you dance through life, let yourself be glad when you find another growing edge. Welcome it: "Oh, I've found another edge, let me accept you." When you feel anger, wonderful! The fire is there to help you. You can trust, 100 percent of the time, that what is in front of you is exactly what you need to embrace. So if you wonder, "Where should I go? Who should I be with? "What should I be doing?", that mental construct—that question itself—is what is separating you from life at that moment. It is the invitation. You are where you need to be, doing what you need to be doing with exactly the right person at exactly this moment. And that is true even if the person you are sitting with right now is "only" you.

If you have any thought at all that carries you away from the full embrace of this nanosecond, there is solidity in that thought that serves as a separating element. This is true whether you are thinking in terms of past, present, or future or in terms of "What should I do, be, or say?" Those constructs keep you separate from the here and now. Embrace possibility in this nanosecond, no exceptions.

You are then the breath of life. You know life to be itself and life to be you, and there is no separation any more. The reason the great masters speak in terms of negatives is that there are no nouns left that you can use to describe yourself. We have only pointer words to say what you are not. You are not what you thought you were. There is no description of what you are, because you are no longer separate.

CHAPTER 5

Forgiveness: the foundation

It has been estimated that greater than eighty percent of all chronic pain has a strong emotional component. With recent data showing a clear correlation between hostility and heart disease, we can no longer ignore the evidence that the hurts, betrayals, and angers we hold close to our heart are, in fact, harming us.

Forgiveness is the portal through which you begin the healing process and enter a deeper state of peace. But forgiveness has often been misidentified. It is not forgiveness when you judge another person and hang on to a sense of self-righteousness and anger. You cannot truly embrace love if you have not forgiven *all* of the past. Forgiveness means deeply embracing everything about your history exactly the way it was. If you have truly forgiven, you do not hold yourself above another, believing yourself to be better or more enlightened because you have "let go" of some atrocious behavior inflicted upon you. Forgiveness means releasing past patterning in every way. It means literally knowing that all is as it should have been and as it should be.

THE PATH TO FORGIVENESS

Although forgiveness is not a linear process, there are recognizable steps or thought processes that lead to true forgiveness, and these are explored in this section.

The first step is to recognize the problem. The problem is probably different than you think it is. If you are angry at another person for what they have done to you, the problem really is the pattern in your own mind that you perceive has been violated by an action outside yourself. If you have a pattern that is so rigid or strict or defined that it could be violated, you are entrapped in an image or illusion of your self. What aggravates one person will not aggravate someone else. Dare to risk discovering what you are holding onto that is so precious. What is the boundary by which you have defined your reality? Whether or not that boundary is agreed upon by society is not at issue here. Recognize it for what it is—a pattern in your own mind.

When you rigidly hold onto a belief, you see everything through a filter. A whole neuronal pattern develops around it, an infrastructure of repeating patterns that is your story. The mildest stimulus can awaken patterning that renders you incapable of hearing through your perceptual field any information that does not support your "reality." You become locked in the castle of your mind, so that whatever a person says will continue to evoke that patterning. This patterning is difficult to break through, but the accomplishment of step one loosens the hold of the whole phenomenon such that success is guaranteed.

To find the patterns of your mind, you must gain within yourself a fundamental desire for honesty and transparency, and a willingness to risk questioning some fundamental "truths" that you have held so dear. You must be willing to accept the possibility that these might be false or that they might not be the only possible interpretation of what is happening. When you drop your defenses to this degree, you have given yourself just enough breathing room so you can step outside that rigid membrane and perhaps begin to glimpse a different possibility. Some of the techniques mentioned in the Appendix, especially meditation, can be extremely helpful in allowing the essential psychic space for this shift to occur. Allow yourself to doubt your own thinking a little bit.

Once you have begun to question your own thinking, you have opened the door to step two. The recognition that whatever you are holding onto is simply a pattern in your mind will lead to a perceptual ripple. You will dare to question the solidity of your perception, and it will no longer be a given. In this step, you will begin to acknowledge those aspects of yourself, your behavior, and your history where you have not been "perfect." If you entertain the question about your perception of yourself and your reality, you will begin a historic review of your own life and your actions. You will not be able to resist it. The whole explanation you have given for everything that has ever happened to you, including your relationships with your parents and family, will come into question. The second step is the hard work you dread, and so it can provide impetus to not bother with the first. It is much easier to maintain a sense that you have forgiven from an aloof space of justified hurt. But that is not forgiveness. True forgiveness requires that you look in the mirror and examine the reflection you see there. In step two you recognize within yourself at least the possibility of those elements you have judged another harshly for.

The third step tends to follow automatically after the second. This is where you are called upon to forgive yourself. Your remedy, ironically, in this entire forgiveness trip is to learn to forgive yourself, but you cannot get to that place if you do not question or let yourself entertain the possibility that you might have done "wrong" or hurtful things to others. This is a very specific definition of forgiveness. It means a deep acceptance of the humanity within you and holding a deep compassion for that humanity. You allow space for an opening into loving kindness. This space is a thing unto itself. It is the in-breath and the out-breath of God, or that infinite space of stillness. It is the Primary Cause that defies definition. It is an absence that is filled with an indefinable presence. It is the absence of fight, the absence of resistance, the absence of judgment, and the absence of antagonism. In the absence of all of these things, you find the pure state of compassion. You greet your Self and welcome in every single facet of your being.

Where there is pain, pause. Do not run away. Drop the story around it. Every single script you are carrying will simply reinforce the pain or explain it to yourself. Rest in the pain. Let it be an invitation to carry your breath and your awareness ever more deeply and into your center. Right there where your pain is the greatest, in the center of your heart, invite peace and loving kindness to enter. Feeling and nourishing your heart this way, from within, allows the pain to be the gateway to surrender into a deeper level of awareness. When you are capable of doing that, you will burst open into the greatest love possible or imaginable, and forgiveness is the inevitable result. When you can forgive from the center of your heart, where the pain is the greatest, no person is capable of hurting you. You have truly surrendered to the divine openness, which is your birthright.

Imagine that your heart is beating with infinite love and wisdom, and hold your focus there. You will probably notice one thing after another—a bit of tension comes up, this or that thought arises. Do not fight it, do not push it away, do not deny it. If you are annoyed, allow that in. Whatever arises, allow your breath to go into it. Invite the in-breath of the heart's fire and energy into whatever arises. No forcing, no fighting. Simply allow. Allow the heart's energy to penetrate whatever arises. Allow every bit of it to come up.

Let go of all the blame, the anger, the resentment. Let go of all of your cherished notions of how you might get back at another person or make them understand. Let go of anything that constricts you, including your self-concept. If you let go of every bit of it, you will rest in a deep and abiding love. In the Bible, John calls this the peace that surpasses all understanding. You move beyond the mind's rationalizations. You "turn the other cheek." You drop the fight because there is no fight to have. Once you have surrendered, there is nothing anyone can do that you would ever again frame as an injury. You will no longer be capable of taking anything personally. You will recognize the hurt and injury that is behind others lashing out, so you are protected in the deepest safety that is possible in this life. As with physical pain, emotional pain is an invitation to surrender into that deep space where there is no need to move and no need to change.

Out of that state of pure compassion, step four organically arises, because wherever you look you will be applying the same principle. That is true forgiveness, in which you accept and embrace the humanity in every person. In this field of compassion you realize that the motivation for every harmful act or speech from anyone (including yourself) has originated from a sense of suffering. That is when you see that there is nothing to forgive. Once again, we are back in the realm of paradox. (You know you are entering a spiritual realm when paradox is the rule!) Once you truly have forgiven, you discover there is nothing to forgive because we are all suffering equally; we are all stuck in this human condition. None of us is any greater than or less than another. We are all just doing the best we can with what we have been able to allow in. Surrender into that deep embrace.

FORGIVENESS AS HEALING

Forgiveness is the only way to free yourself from the past and open the portal to a different future. As you embrace the greater fullness of yourself, without justification or defenses, you step closer to living your true potential. *This* is living life to the fullest. Beyond the concepts of disease versus wellness, you begin to embark on a whole new adventure.

Through absolute forgiveness there is not one iota of anything left in you that holds the desire to harm or to get back in any way. Not one thread of resentment is left when you have surrendered in this place completely. You are incapable of doing harm. The energy from this space will influence your neuronal network so that your thinking will follow different patterns. It is the magnetic impulse that literally recalibrates your mind's functioning. You will rework your history, your past, and your future. Your mind will operate differently, and it will be motivated by the heart's impulse. You will have evolved into a different state of being. You will know yourself to be absolutely safe. That is because *you are* the impulse of love, you are the impulse of life, and you are always perpetually safe. You will be delivered to a place where you experience no more wounding, no hurt, no pain, and no suffering.

When you find yourself in this space of being, a sense of graciousness and gratitude marks your behavior. You will recognize each encounter as a blessing. Every breath is marked by gratitude in simply living, and every interaction fosters forgiveness in the moment. There is no residue, nothing that you hang onto. Everything is as it is, and you are filled with a simple awareness of being.

CHAPTER 6

Love: the heart of the matter

Love is an interesting phenomenon. You might think of love as something you get from another person or that is somehow attached to and associated with a person, place, or situation. But the reality is that you do not *get* love or *create* love, love awakens in you. Love is revealed to your awareness by dropping constriction. It is a physiologic, tangible, organic space of being, and it centers in the heart. When you drop the shackles of fear, your innate state of being reveals itself, and you resonate with that essence.

If you have experienced heartache and heartbreak, you know the unique misery that is experienced when you have made an effort toward love and it has been thwarted in some way. When that happens, you might stop in your tracks and surround your heart with bitterness to shield or anesthetize yourself against the agony of what you are feeling. But that is an invitation to sorrow and disease, because you have constricted your energy. Love, accessed through forgiveness, is the cure.

The love impulse may lead you along a path that makes no sense to the thinking mind. The heart is ultimately greater than the mind, however, and will have its way with you. You can trust that if you have been propelled into a situation by love, it will take you right to the threshold of where your deepest limitation to love currently exists. You may feel that limitation in the form of pain. Sometimes the source of that pain will come through the voice, the gestures, and the energy of a person you are with, and sometimes it is contained within your own mind, but you can count on the fact that if love has been the impulse—no matter how you define that love or characterize it—the situations you are drawn to will lead you into the invitation to forgive if you have experienced pain in association with it. You will find yourself magnetized to situations that allow deep healing to occur.

We all have a boundary beyond which we deny the existence of love or are unable to take it in. As we have explored, you believe there is some part of you that is so abhorrent you cannot imagine love penetrating there. That defines your place of pain. So if you are delivered to that place, recognize it as your own constriction inviting you into a greater opening. The agony of the thwarted love impulse is the most severe pain of which humans are capable because it emanates from the center of the heart. It is the heart calling you home. In Chinese medicine, the heart energy is referred to as fire, and sooner or later you will be immersed in that fire. The heart opens when you are completely surrendered into that state of being that is beyond definition. This is the true state of love.

IMPEDIMENTS TO THE AWARENESS OF LOVE

As you progress along this path, you will undoubtedly experience certain impediments to your progress. These are the last bits and pieces that will hold you captive and keep you from surrendering. Your own resistance is the only real impediment, but it takes many forms. It is useful to be aware of the signposts that indicate you are in resistance so that perhaps you will not be seduced by them quite so frequently. If you are to release the myriad images that you believe identify you, you must notice the ways your self-image is threatened. This is the classic domain of the ego. The ego arises when you define yourself by anything other than the free flow of life. You must drop anything at all in life that you cling to or resist, anything that comes at you, anything that threatens your self definition, any defenses you harbor—you must drop it all.

A common impediment is self-doubt, or doubt in what may be possible. Doubt is recognizable as an inner sense of pause, the last backward glance, the "what if" questions: "What if this is not true?" "What if I'm making this up?" "What if I will be lied to again or betrayed again?" Well, what if you surrender and find out what is on the other side?! What have you got to lose but the past?

Another impediment is the self-aggrandizement you experience in insisting that you are a separate self. You have so many variations on this. As odd as this may sound, you need your misery in order to define yourself as separate and therefore important. You must give up your attachment to the separate self, which will, paradoxically, release your sense of suffering. It is so simple, but admittedly hard to do.

Guilt is another impediment. You may fear that perhaps you truly have done something wrong to deserve the misery you are experiencing. Unfortunately, this is played upon by religions that use guilt as a method of power and control. Perhaps it is nobly motivated, but nonetheless it is faulty thinking and is an impediment to surrender.

A close analog of guilt is shame. Shame is a distorted sense of self. At some level it is the insistence that you do not deserve to exist. Sometimes this shame masquerades as humility, but it is still ego. Shame is not the way you get rid of ego—in fact, you do not *get rid of* ego at all—ego is the fight you are having. Just let it go. When you drop the fight, the ego no longer exists. The only thing that keeps the ego alive is the fight that you engage in by looking for the "problem." Those of you who are perpetual seekers and self-analyzers might pause to unearth and uproot the last of your impediments— the tendency to constantly define one more thing that you might need to let go of or get rid of. *It is the searching for what is wrong with you that keeps you stuck.* Love does not need you to sort through your whole knapsack. Just set it down. Cross over the brink and surrender. Love's invitation is whole and complete, and is waiting to welcome you *as you are*. That is the irony—you do not need to be anything different from what you are right now.

For those who have been seeking for a long time, a question that might arise is, "Why am I not 'there' yet?" You intellectually understand what is necessary to cross the threshold into a new way of being, but you question why, if it is really possible to do so, you haven't actuated yet. This is again one of those slippery slopes. It is the language of doubt. Recognize it for what it is and do not be seduced. It is like saying, "If I am capable of being five feet tall, why must I be 4 foot 8?" Because you are young, and you are growing into it! So relax where you are. Take this breath in, and invite the heart energy to where you are now. You have more to allow through you, that is all. It is a process, and wherever you are is okay.

Another impediment might be the fear of being different or the fear of being punished in some way. You contain the karmic remembrance of historic tragedies such as burning witches, the holocaust and other human atrocities, and you might be acutely aware of how society tends to marginalize those who are "different." If you have been set apart or in any way defined as superior in a frightening sort of way, you may fear being punished, criticized, or harmed if you reveal a deeper knowing. It is highly unlikely that you will have to experience crucifixion or burning at the stake, but the cultural memory and the fear of those possibilities may resonate in your being. The martyr archetype signified by such karmic memories is prevalent, particularly in the Western world, so that fear is very real for you. Shrouded around that fear are layers of guilt and shame for many of you, because you have personalized the hatred that was flung at you. This again is an invitation to surrender into forgiveness at the deepest level. Jesus demonstrated through his crucifixion on the cross how you must be willing to recognize the innocence of even those who have harmed you the most. That recognition must be sincere and legitimate right down to the very core of your being. Surrender the fear itself. Do not give up wisdom for the sake of protecting yourself at that depth. You contain within yourself all the archetypes. Do not confuse those archetypal energies as a personal problem. When you have deeply surrendered, that fear will be nonexistent.

Judgment is a major impediment to love. It is time to move beyond dualism and polarity and recognize that judgment is at the root of many of your problems. If you judge another being, or any aspect of another being, you have judged yourself, because you contain within yourself every element of life's potential. If you deny the cruelty that is contained within your potentiality, you are denying your inherent being. You must take equal responsibility, along with every other living being, for life as it has played out thus far. Count on the fact that *anything* you judge harshly in someone else reflects that element within yourself that you are not acknowledging. You must claim and deeply accept within the fabric of your being those elements that you most abhor in others. Allow the sensations to play out inside yourself and do not resist. What you resist in another—including ignoring or denying—you are resisting in yourself. Herein lies your greatest work. When you love that scar which most needs your attention and develop the capacity to accept your shadow pieces, the compassion gushes out of your heart like a great geyser. It embraces those around you with such enormous empathy that the resonance shifts your entire structure. This cannot be emphasized enough, because there is such a profound need for this type of acceptance now. It is an immense healing force.

This does not mean you stand by permissively while watching harm being done. Ironically, that is a lack of acceptance. That is a tensing up in constriction around your capacity to do what is most needed in response to what is in front of you. The idea of victimization (regarding yourself or someone else) invites the perpetrator and visa versa. To the extent that you deeply accept, you will know the perfect words to say or action to take to appease the situation and reduce the cruelty that has come into your experience. Eventually you will come to see the innocence in the other, even if you were the target of malicious behavior designed to hurt. You will know that behind every angry gesture is a hurting soul.

It does not work to try to pretend you are at this stage before you really are. You first must attend to yourself in a responsible way. People do cause harm, so being gentle and kind to yourself is of paramount importance.

Ironically, another possible impediment to surrendering to love is the fear that there will be nothing to do if you have no problems. Embrace the possibility that if you live with full and complete gratitude, you will have plenty to do. You will be imbued by a grace and dignity spawned from the most enormous wealth of energy you can imagine. Gratitude is an energy force that nourishes and feeds love. When you make this connection, the cycle is complete and self-sustaining. Every moment you awaken with gratitude in your heart, it spawns the next act of love, which continues the gratitude. To the extent you allow yourself to continue surrendering breath by breath, moment by moment, you will be continually infused with the energy of gratitude. You will be grateful for *every* situation you encounter. You will feel grateful for the pain and life's tough situations because you recognize everything that happens provides an opportunity to in-fill that circumstance with greater love. What greater work is there?

So you will not be bored. There is plenty to do when you are filled with love and compassion. It will not leave you problem-free, but your problems become simply situations in which you find yourself. Grace will guarantee that you will always be in the right place at the right time—you always are anyway, but you will know it to be true. You will experience infinite trust dwelling in your heart that spawns deep relaxation. You will no longer try to "figure out" what you should do, what you should say, where you should be, or what you should do with your life, because you are letting life do with you what it needs done. The way you spend your energy is profoundly different and indeed you have much energy to spend. This is not the superficial, Pollyannaish, nice-guy/nice-girl syndrome, where there is always a bit of irritation underneath it all or a sense of dependency upon a particular behavior to be accepted. Once you have deeply accepted every facet of life, life will have accepted every facet of you. Life becomes your best friend.

It takes only this moment to surrender to love. Many of you are actually in the transitory phase, moving in and out of awareness. You understand the truth of what is being said here. The final surrender requires vigilance around these final impediments so you can recognize them for what they are and let go.

ROMANTIC LOVE

Mental constructs are addictive patterns within your neuronal network. These patterns result in familiar sensations which, even if they are painful, can bring a certain level of comfort because they are familiar. Any effort to make behavioral or circumstantial change is superficial at best unless you pause long enough to go into the sensations themselves. You must rest there and recognize the addiction contained in those sensations.

What we tend to call romantic "love" actually is not love at all, but a sense of deep familiarity and therefore comfort. It creates a sense of safety that gives you permission to open up into the love that you are immersed in all the time. However, most of us project the source of love onto the other person, and then it becomes a syrupy state of affairs, where you want either to get something from the other person or to rescue them so you can feel needed. What is actually motivating you in these cases is a deep sense of being unlovable. When you perceive yourself to be "falling in love," you are actually opening deeply at the cellular level into the sensation of possibility. It is more accurate to say that you have fallen into a state of grace in which your cells open up to receive the love that is always available. In that moment, you embrace the breath of life and love in which you are immersed.

The resonance that is created when you encounter another and embrace possibility opens you up to that which is always there. Heartbreak occurs when you clench down into the constriction of a faulty belief—the belief that losing love is possible. All suffering is contained within your own mind. To the extent that you can surrender into love as an *a priori* state—your natural state of being—you will not be afraid of loss in the way you are now.

So what is relationship all about? When you are attracted to someone—romantically or otherwise—you activate a mental construct. When someone resonates in a familiar pattern, you feel a mix of comfort and excitement. You open to possibility. You understand and are finally understood and it is beautiful. However, sooner or later, love will magnify your mental constructs and crack you open into a deeper awareness of hidden pain. You will most likely project the problem onto the other person, just as you projected the love onto the other person. Until you wake up to the idea that it is the pattern itself that needs your attention, you will fight. You will want everything outside you to change to make your life less miserable. You will want that person to love you more, to make you feel better. But it cannot work that way.

It is quite normal to experience sadness when you have invested a lot of yourself in a particular person, place or situation that disappears from your daily life. You will undoubtedly experience a sensation in the body when that happens. But if you have identified this "other" as the *source* of your comfort, you will likely cave in around it, and then it becomes pathological.

The tendency we all have when we find ourselves in uncomfortable situations is to flee into the notion of "Oh, I made a mistake" or "There is something wrong with that other person" or "This is a recurring pattern." Indeed, it will be a recurring pattern until you surrender! This does not mean you surrender into abuse. It means the healing cannot occur until you fully accept the person or situation *as it is*. You surrender—or let go of—your resistance, and allow yourself to be in love with "what is." Sometimes the person with whom you are involved will be propelled into a healing with you, but there is no guarantee about that. There may come a time when you must let go of a particular form. Do not be attached to forms. Whether you leave the relationship or stay with it, you will understand that the other is completely innocent. You are both always completely innocent. From the attached perspective, the way you characterize or define the other is through the filter of your own fear or anger, so you often mishear and misinterpret whatever is said or done. This is precisely what leads you to the greater awareness of your own patterns, to the extent you remain open to this learning.

Love is never lost to you. You simply no longer have a particular experience of relationship. Every year, the leaves fall and the trees lose their leaves, and that is just how it is. Every interaction, every phenomenon, every experience you ever have in life will come and go—it is natural. Let yourself get used to the sensation of loss and do not allow yourself to convert it into pathology. This requires trust. It requires deep surrender into the heart. When you recognize that you are love and therefore you cannot lose it, you experience the safety to be open-hearted in every situation. You will no longer fear losing people. You will fill the space around you with the awareness of love, and others will respond to that energy.

Love is not outside you. It is not a package that one person gives to another. It is the life that flows through you. In the womb, you existed within embryonic fluid, and that same fluid continually coursed through your veins. Similarly, love is that "embryonic fluid" in which you float. It is that life from which you originate, which maintains you, and which dances the molecules in every breath you take. It is the energy within which you are immersed and that you completely contain. You are never separate from love. You cannot be unloved—it is the condition of being human and being alive. You must remember this and stop looking to a form to "find" love. You are love manifesting itself, waiting to wake up to itself.

CHAPTER 7

Peace: your essential state

Peace is an essential state that reflects our fundamental character. It is our natural state of being when all fighting has ceased. No external circumstance is needed to develop peace—you need do nothing to establish it. We hear such a cry for peace in the world today because we each have an enormously deep longing to return to that essential state. Your task is to recognize the many ways you keep the fight going, and take personal responsibility for every bit of it. Until you do, peace is only a mental concept.

As we have been discussing, divisive energy originates from your mental constructs—your thoughts. You return to peace when you recognize yourself as trapped within these mental constructs. You are then able to increase your capacity to embrace and see beyond these stuck mind patterns. It is possible to increasingly live your life from a state of internal harmony wherein conflict does not guide your decisions, reactions, behavior, or even your thoughts.

As in the story of Adam and Eve, conflict begins with the recognition of good and evil. From that point, you are locked in to seeing right/wrong, either/or, this/that, good/bad. When your perceptual focus shifts to see one aspect or the other, you cannot see the whole. Adam and Eve recognized the self as separate, automatically birthing a sense of polarity. If there is a "self," there must be a "not self." When you move beyond a sense of the separate self as the defining factor of your life, you can no longer do harm to any being, any creature, or any facet of the earth without recognizing the harm that is done to yourself. That is the spiritual kernel to which you are being invited to return.

Defining "good" and "bad" in rigid delineations automatically sets up the fight mentality. Unfortunately, many religions use judgment to define the "correct" way of being and living in the world. When you think of the millions of people who have been killed in the name of religious beliefs, you will see how flawed that thinking must be at its base. Ironically, many "peacemakers" or "peaceworkers" contain within themselves the very elements of conflict they are trying to alleviate. To the extent this internal conflict continues, the fight continues. As long as you are immersed in the addictive pattern of conflict, even if you lay aside your physical weapons, the internal strife continues to manifest in other ways. The internal tension keeps you from seeing that you are engaged in a battle. While polarities exist in your mind, you are always in conflict, although you may be harnessing that conflictual energy in more "new age" or genteel fashion.

You must search within yourself for disagreements—those places where you are holding onto a particular point of reference. It is not at all uncommon to contain two opposing points of reference within yourself, and vary the details of how they play out from one relationship to another. For example, how often have you had the experience of playing a particular part in a scenario or conversation and then shortly thereafter discover you are playing the opposite part? To the extent that you can wake up to that fact, you can embrace the whole. Living in this state of paradox allows room for the apparent polarities to exist without causing you to get caught in the energy pattern of competition.

The inner essence of the yin yang symbol depicts this dynamic. Yin and yang constantly flow into each other. One cannot be dispelled in the face of the other. In fact, it is impossible to get rid of either, because the opposites are interdependent within the whole and define one another by their mutual existence. So it is that when you embrace polarities simply as mutually dependent elements and drop the internal pattern of tension and resistance against any one part of it, you will be on track.

In other words, what is needed to return to the essential state of peace is to drop all resistance. As discussed earlier, dropping resistance is not the same as "giving in," because giving in implies that there is still some element against which you have no power. As long as you have a sense of needing to give in to something like pain, anger, or a difficult situation, you are fighting. Dropping resistance means attaining a large enough vision that it is possible to embrace the polarities through awareness of them.

MENTAL CONSTRUCTS AS OBSTACLES TO PEACE

Your mental constructs have many variations. They are like tinker toys in your mind—easily assembled and deconstructed. In particular, there are many subtle variations of blame. When you look for an explanation of life circumstances by anybody or anything outside you, you are blaming. Stop looking outward for the basis of the reality you are experiencing. You are simply having an experience. Stop blaming and rest right in the middle of your experience. Notice the fight. Can you see what a dreadful waste it is to be fighting with anything outside yourself? It is as if someone has their hand on your forehead and you are swinging at them like crazy, or like you are banging your head on a wall that will not give. It is all happening in your imagination.

Stop right where you are and embrace whatever is happening. You are where you are by your own thinking. That is a very powerful idea, because it means you can change it. Welcome the opportunity to wake up to what is inside, right where you are. Blaming yourself does no good, either. It is still a way of not being completely responsible. It is a contraction against what is. Nobody, including yourself, is at fault. The "fault" is in the perceptual framework, which is created by your sense of yourself as separate.

• *The Heart of Healing* •

Your perceptual framework is like the eye trying to see itself, which is why it is so difficult. Because the eye cannot see itself, the world is your mirror. The problem is that when you are confused, you scrub the mirror like crazy, thinking that will solve the perceived problems. That does not work. Instead of trying to wipe the mirror when you look and see a smudge on your nose, reach up and touch your nose. Look at it. Feel it. Do not blame the mirror, which is just reflecting your perceptual framework back to you, and do not blame yourself, because you just got confused.

Anger is an interesting energy—a forceful, powerful, delightful energy. It is the fire that can burn dross if you allow it to. You learn to feel your anger more completely when you drop resistance entirely and allow it to flow through you as the fire that it is. By feeling it in your body without fighting, it passes through and helps you awaken to your mental constructs.

It is essential, however, that you not allow your anger to walk through the path of blame. To engage your anger energy along the path of blame can do harm to yourself and to others. It is a method of keeping yourself engaged fruitlessly, going around in circles and dragging others along with you, if they are susceptible. It is an engagement of a construct that becomes even more complex if you do not own it. Anger through the path of blame keeps people confused because there tends to be a lot of reactivity against it. That is why it is so important to recognize every facet of yourself that is doing the blame trip.

Taking full responsibility for your mental patterns and for the anger energy itself means you allow yourself to feel it completely and let the purity of the energy burn right through. That may mean you speak clearly and succinctly and without apology, owning your feelings and taking full responsibility for them. It may mean that you request change, but it will be from a clean, clear space—not from blame.

As mentioned earlier, fear is also a component of a predominant mental construct and is a primary obstacle to peace. It is like a skein of yarn wrapped so tightly around the heart of the matter that you think of it as your identity. It is punctuated by nuances, and it is tricky and slippery. Because it is the innermost layer wrapped around the core from which you fight the most intensely, surrendering while in a state of fear is the deepest place of surrender.

For example, if you are fearful of not being liked, you hold an inner tension around this fear. You attempt to make yourself likeable to overcome this hidden kernel of fear, but the effort itself creates an energy that either repulses individuals or hooks them into some sort manipulative framework that is not quite comfortable for either of you. You develop a whole lifestyle, a whole network of friends, a whole series of activities with this hidden kernel as the foundation, and that kernel gets further and further away from your awareness.

To surrender into the deep acceptance of yourself in the midst of this profound sensation is a final act of true surrender. You are no longer running from yourself—from that which you fear the most. When you drop the fight based on your fear of fear, you have come home.

FINDING THE PEACE WITHIN

The rule is the same no matter where you are along the path: stop fighting what is. On the outermost layer, stop fighting your life circumstances, or whatever predicament you find yourself in. Imagine in this very moment that there are no mistakes about your life as it is. Decide: "I am here by choice to awaken to some reality in my own mental construct." Embrace this idea with curiosity, asking, "What is this, here where I am? What is the special gift I have given myself in this life circumstance? What am I here to awaken to?"

Now go deeply into the next layer, your feelings. What sensations do you feel in your body right here where you are? Do not fight anything. Settle down into your body in this one circumstance. Do not explain, analyze, try to figure it out, or review the circumstance. Just settle in and feel it. Feel it deeply. Drop every bit of anesthesia, such as food, alcohol, caffeine, or busyness. Drop anything that alters your mental framework and keeps you from feeling.*

Instead of judging or resisting anything or anyone, rest quietly and observe what is going on. Notice the polarities without feeling compelled to tense up in defense against one belief in the name of the other. For example, if you believe that one can only be a "good" person when free of greed or anger, you set yourself up for failure when you experience any such "bad" emotion. And denying that you are caught in such an internal fight guarantees that the conflict will reflect itself in your relationships. You will project it onto others. Although projection is a psychological term, it is rooted in spiritual fact.

Allow yourself to honestly feel what you are and where you are. As you enter into the feeling, notice the internal fight, which might be something like, "But I don't want to feel pain." Welcome it in as if you are inviting it to sit with you at the table. Ask, "What is this?" Develop an intense curiosity. As each sensation comes along ask again, "What is this?" Layer after layer after layer of mental constructs will come to the surface as you do this very simple, profound practice. Every time you allow thoughts, emotions and sensations to effortlessly bubble up, and you welcome them without resisting, they evaporate on their own. Anything on which you shine your direct, unobstructed line of vision, with clarity and without fight, dissolves into its truest nature. The falsehoods will melt away and the true gem you have longed for will surface.

As you sit with your life circumstances, you will probably learn that you have been doing all sorts of things that are not true to yourself in order to make yourself likeable. You are doing this to overcome an inherent deficiency that only you "know." It is your little secret. So recognize that as the place to make true, deep change in your life. Start to get more honest with yourself. Feel in your body how you do not like your life circumstances. The first thing that will likely come to the surface is resistance. Allow it in. Embrace it.

Eventually, you may find yourself having less need to lie to someone in order to fit in or be liked. You may begin to be more careful

---

* I am not recommending that you go off prescribed drugs if you need them, but do understand that it is part of the anesthesia. Start where you are.

about what you agree to and what you say to different people and who you feel legitimately attracted to. As you go deeper, you will come to some place inside that is shimmering with the worst pain of all. You may get in touch with a painful childhood memory, such as the first time you perceived you were not liked. Stay with it and pay attention. That sensation has defined your whole reality up to this point. You must rest without resistance in the middle of this horribly painful feeling. You must go there, because that is where you will finally experience the complete undoing of the world as you know it. The only way out is to go back through that emotional scar.

Do this without questioning where it came from. Do not analyze. Analysis is a way to keep yourself from surrendering into it by keeping you in your head. Embrace yourself wherever you find yourself to be—do not run away from it. You must *feel* it. Only then will it evolve and melt away. For a while you may feel annihilated, because your whole reality has been based around this flaw—it is the prism that locks in your entire world view. But this is the call to your own beloved life. It is your life that is on the other side of the chasm awaiting your recognition.

Everything you have read and all you have been taught are simply pointers and explanations from those who have traversed the path before you. Learning more words about it will not make any difference. None of it will save you from having to walk the path of your own body and your own life. There is no way around it. It is hard work, and nobody can do it for you.

Let your breath explain the reality of your existence on the planet. Pay attention to its essence. It is both inside you and outside you—it comes in and goes out. It represents the molecular structure of everything around you. You cannot own your breath. You call it "your" breath, but how long is it "your" breath? You breathe out, and it is gone! It does not belong to you. It is the same with "your own" life—it does not belong to you, either. What "belongs" to "you" is the craziness, the mental constructs. Let them become fluid. Let yourself be life attempting to experience itself in all its multi-faceted beauty. We all share breath and we all share the one life.

PEACE MEDITATION

The following meditation is designed to help you find the love you are and bring you peace. Read it through, and then set the book down and allow it to organically unfold.

>Imagine that you have no name. Just sit with that idea for awhile.
>
>Now imagine that you have no story—no story about who you are, where you are, who is with you, what you do, how you do it—no story at all.
>
>All you have is the breath in and the breath out.
>
>Open your eyes and look around you.
>
>Realize that all you have is right in front of you.
>
>This moment is what you have. And now that moment gone—and only this moment. Always this moment.
>
>There is nothing to do, nowhere to go that is any different from where you are.
>
>Drop your judgment. Allow it all to be, and embrace it.
>
>Now sit and watch your breath. Let it come in, let it go out.
>
>Let your breath be whatever it is.
>
>Just as you hang on to no breaths, hang on to no moments.
>
>Hang on to no view, no attitude.
>
>Hang on to nothing.
>
>Things define your reality only to the extent that you are entrapped in your mind. Let the fluidity be what defines you.
>
>As you look around in this surrendered state, you will see everything around you vibrating with life energy, with love. You will know how infinitely safe you are.
>
>With every breath in and every breath out, live in the awareness of yourself as that love. That is who you are.
>
>You are life trying to experience itself as love. That is the longing you have for connection. It is the longing you have to move beyond separation.

Wake up. Know who you really are.

Love is calling you back home.

You can trust that the impulse of love will guide you correctly.

All healing happens from the state of love.

This is peace.

CHAPTER 8

Soul: the portal to peace

You might think about owning a soul as if it were an individual possession. You may recognize that your biological entity is temporary, and think of the soul as a part of you that continues after your physical death. But you are not a body walking around with a soul, or even a soul with a body. Soul can be viewed as the aperture into another dimension. On earth, we tend to think of ourselves as individual, discrete entities. As we settle into soul awareness, we enter a space of knowing in which there are not singular entities as you think of yourself. In the three-dimensional realm, your karmic imprints are contained within an energy pattern you call your self. As you move through the aperture of the soul, you will remember that you are not an individual, separate self. Soul is your portal back to that awareness.

Look at an open door. Notice that the doorjamb—the solid frame—is not the doorway. The doorway is the space, or the portal, through which you walk to get to the other side. Likewise, the soul is not a solid thing. It is the spaciousness through which life experiences itself, coming and going. It is a space where apparently disparate polarities can comfortably co-exist. This is why we experience paradox as a "norm" here.

PAIN AS AN ACCESS POINT

If soul is the doorway, you might view pain as one possible doorknob. It can be seen as a means of entering the doorway to the deeper awareness of soul Contained within the fabric of your physical structure—your DNA coding—is the energetic quality of all the archetypes and familial history into which you were born. These patterns pull you into their working matrix over and over again until you start to wake up to their existence. The good news is that this apparently solid structure of "what is" is only a figment of the mind. By changing your mind, you change the entire scene, including past, present, and future. It all happens in exactly this moment—the one you are in. Thereby, and only thereby, can you change your reality and your future. Otherwise, you continue to replay the encoding into which you were born.

You are misled to the extent that you define pain only as an error in your thinking rather than recognizing it for the deep gift it is. Strive less to get rid of pain and realize that it is simply the messenger. Use it to gain access to a deeper dimension of yourself. Pain will "magically" disappear as your old structure, your old way of being, and your explanation of being shift and change. Your relationships and everything in your body can be different. You will then have a different experience of yourself.

To change yourself at such a fundamental level will naturally invoke structural upheaval. At times you may feel like you are dying, and you will be in some sense. The sensations of this dying may seem unendurable, and in fact they are because the structure of your self as you know it will not endure. It is a biological fact that you will not be the same. The familiar is comfortable in its own way, and many would rather remain in pain and chaos than go through such a change. You perceive great risk in daring to dissolve your structures so deeply, because on the other side of it you will no longer be who you now know yourself to be. But that is the "death" you must endure. Only in dying can you be born again—not in the "name of Christ," or in the name of anything outside yourself, but in the name of the free flow of energy you can access when you allow yourself to dissolve the DNA/karmic imprint with which you are familiar.

Many people awaken through a horrific insult to their sentient being. A great illumination can happen to those who, for example, have a terminal illness or serious emotional or physical pain, or a crisis that rips the fabric of their lives completely away from them. When everything you held dear is taken away, you can experience profound moments when you recognize your true Self. An increasing number of people in the world are suffering at such a depth, and many eventually drop it all and walk across the threshold to awakening. If you are in such pain, that is what you are being called to do. The pain will not be with you forever. You will have sensations as long as you have a body, but you will never again see it the same once you have completely surrendered to the greater depth of who you really are.

HUMANS AS THE PARADOX

Humans are in a fascinating, precarious predicament. Standing in the open doorway of soul awareness, you can maintain cognitive awareness of yourself as an individual simultaneous to recognizing your connection to the whole of life. No other life form can do this. Other life forms play out their part blissfully and fully and completely. They do not question. But you *are* the question, the incarnate paradox. You are the element of life itself coming and going. You have the capacity for it all—suffering and bliss. To the extent that you are open, you allow life to fully flow through you, and you get to have the awareness of it.

Pain seems very real when you are stuck in it, of course, but when you allow life's breath to move through you, you will no longer be able to define any life experience as pain. Pain is not the truth, and suffering is a mental pattern that can be changed. You can let go of the notion that suffering is necessary. Similarly, true forgiveness is the recognition that there is nothing to forgive. This is your natural state. As your facades, habits, and patterns thin out and become transparent, you simply observe it all and laugh, because you *are* it all. You do not cling because you know you are the open door. You are in that place where you absolutely know there is no separation. You will feel infinite peace vibrating through every cell of your body and truly know, experientially, that all is well.

Love every facet of life. Love even your resistance. From this place of peace, no harm can be done to you or by you. You know that every act of life is simply a nuance of the dance. When you exist in this love, you are no longer afraid. The shadow is gone and you exist in a place of pure light. Life completely has its way with you, and you have no resistance left. Life is "what is."

This is how the world as we know it ends. Those who are awake will experience the new world—it is a matter of awareness. Yes, there will be destruction, and that is okay, because it will be the destruction of old forms. It is natural that they fall away.

YOUR SOUL'S PURPOSE

You may have heard that you should strive to fulfill your soul's purpose. Instead, allow your soul's purpose to find you. Surrender your individual will, not to something that is separate or controlling you, but into that space where you know yourself not to be separate. You can resonate with life that the soul, as a portal, can provide to and through you. You might experience this as heaven.

Heaven is not a separate place you go to. It is that experience of being from which you originated and to which you long to return. Words cannot begin to describe it. As you allow infinite peace to resonate through your structure, your language and your way of being will reflect that heaven more deeply. As you rest there, you will feel the energy vibration of your body emanating love.

To experience heaven, you must commit to having the heart open exactly where you are at any moment—no exceptions. Then you truly are the portal. You bring the essence of yourself into the world fully and completely, and *that* is what you are called to do and to be. That is your purpose. Allow your body to be fully lit with the soul's energy, which means allowing the light of the infinite to flow through you. You will begin to recognize the face of the beloved in every facet of life you encounter. You will recognize that everything you see is a reflection of yourself.

You are the breath of life. You are the fluidity. You are the perpetual movement of what you may call God. You are infinity encapsulated in form. You are love.

CHAPTER 9

Returning home: the dance

This book has offered suggestions about how to invite the dance of life into the whole of your being, into the cells of your physical structure, and return home to peace. Let's review how to embrace your mindbody as the path to spiritual awakening.

As we have explored, if you experience tension or pain, it is an indication that there is a fight going on. You are in some way saying "no" to what is. Practice saying "yes" to everything, including your resistance. Whatever your experience is, just smile and say "yes." Try it for a day, and see what transforms. If you find resistance in yourself and you get upset because you have resistance, you begin building layers of tension. When you let go of resistance, the tension melts away, pain decreases and you find yourself to be content with what is. New possibilities paradoxically can reveal themselves to you in this ease, so if change is called for it can more easily happen.

Where you feel tense, invite the breath of life. Imagine that you embrace what is right in front of you, as if it were a friend here to tell you something. Drop the resistance to your immediate experience—as you are feeling it right now—in your mindbody. Above all, try not to project. It is helpful to recognize that every facet of your life experience is an expert mirror to help you along your journey. If you think anything is outside you, pause and reflect upon it as a shadow you are casting through your own resistance. Never doubt

The Heart of Healing

for a second but that you are in the right place at the right time, interacting with the right person. There are no exceptions and no mistakes about where you are or with whom you are interacting, there is only your interpretation of it and what you do with it. That does not mean, by the way, that you should take accusations levied at you at face value—not at all. It does mean that your interactions and reactions are giving you material to work with, providing potential for your gradual awakening.

Every situation stimulates experiential sensations in addition to interpretations of the phenomenon. Question your interpretations, and rest ever more deeply in the sensations themselves. Let your body guide you to where life is inviting you to the dance. Remember, you are life. Life is you. You are your experience—*all* of it. You are the complete harmonic, and the experience of you includes the restriction(s). You are the life pattern playing itself out. There are no exceptions and there are no mistakes. Rest in that knowing. Be your own best friend. Whatever feeling or experience you have, be oh so deeply gentle and kind. You will not like some experiences, and it is here that it is especially important to be kind. Pause and invite the light right into the tension, so that every cell of your body can vibrate with the life that is seeking its expression through you and as you. Let yourself vibrate with joy.

In this culture, one of our primary reactions to anything uncomfortable is to anesthetize ourselves. We want more than anything to just not experience discomfort at all. We do not even want to know anything about it, so we try very hard to numb out. The second thing we want to do is blame, so we find the fault "out there." We go to great lengths to change whomever we are with to make ourselves more comfortable—to clean the face of the mirror, so to speak. We also focus on trying to change ourselves. This may sound odd, but that is not the answer either. The point is not to try to change ourselves. The point is to rest deeply within the awareness of our true Self, which is beyond the awareness of our false beliefs.

Do not try to *do* anything. Do not run away. Do not fight with the other, and do not fight with yourself.

Your teacher is with you every moment of your life as the experience you are having. In accepting this, you have moved beyond the paradigm of needing a guru, which can be part of a storyline. It is helpful sometimes to be with a person who does exactly the right thing at exactly the right time to help you wake up in that moment. But as you encounter life itself as your teacher, you begin to recognize every face in front of you as a teacher in that moment. Then your teacher is with you every second—you can never get away from your teacher.

Question what you think of as reality. When you have a thought about something that occurred, about somebody else, or about yourself, ask yourself, "Is this true? Is it *really* true?" Dare to hold yourself in that open space of curiosity. Give yourself permission to experience what your life might be like without the fight. Another helpful question is, "What if I just accepted this?" Sink into the sensations in your body. Ask, "What if this moment is just perfect the way it is?" That is really a safe question, because if the answer is illuminating you have gained a great deal—if it is not, you can always revert to your former position. Increasingly, you will realize that, of course, this moment is perfect as it is because it quite simply could not possibly be different. Each moment is the natural consequence of all the preceding moments leading up to it, and could not be other than what it is. Acceptance of this truth is deeply transformative. In that breath, you realize that making the choice of being totally present—in compassion, in acceptance—is precisely that which defines the trajectory of your future. That transforming moment can only happen *now*.

Other stretching questions include: "What if the opposite of what I think is true is true?" "What if what that person said to me that pushed all my buttons was a fact?" "What if the criticism I'm struggling against is actually true for me?" "What if I try on that thought?" No harm is done in just trying it on. Ask with sincerity as a receptacle into which the answer is invited to be revealed. When you ask questions as a rhetorical device, a defensive stance, you are not going to get very far. You will know the difference. If you still experience tension and fight, then you didn't mean the question as a sincere question.

Every bit of resistance must eventually fall away—any effort to make anything different than it is. This means letting go of any sense of how you or someone else should appear when you are "spiritual." If you feel disdain or discomfort or unhappiness because you or someone else has not yet "arrived," that too is the fight mentality. That fight energy creates an inner tension and resistance to the flow of life as it is. So the secret is to drop *all* judgments and move beyond the polarities of right/wrong or good/bad. Accept exactly what is in front of you or within you. When you do that, the first thing that arises is love.

It is quite egotistical, isn't it, to think that it is our effort that makes the difference? That is exactly what we are waking up to when we drop the ego. The ego is not something to fight or get rid of. When we drop the fight, the ego itself disappears because *the ego is that sense of separation that is created by having the fight and the resistance against "what is."* The ego is that membrane against which we fight, which gives us a self-identity. That is what you are disbanding by making no effort, so it is actually quite pain free.

You think the great sacrifice is to get rid of the familiar, but the problem really is your fear and dread and the fight you create about letting it go. Compare that situation to how your immune system reacts to an allergen. The immune system gets hyper-excited, fighting against the perceived pathogen. But the allergen is not a pathogen at all, it is simply something your system will not allow in. The warfare that ensues is completely confined within your immune system. Ironically, all the chemicals your immune system dumps out causes harm to your tissue. Every symptom you have from an allergic reaction is your own immune system gone amok and fighting itself.

In our culture today, our immune systems are over-activated. We are all in fight mode. There is a war pretty much on everything—war on drugs, war on terrorism, war on war. We are all deeply allergic to life these days, and our autoimmune systems are fighting ourselves. We manifest inside the personal body exactly what we see outside ourselves, and vice versa. Again, the secret of it all is to drop the fight. Stop believing you can fight war with war.

We are in quite a state of affairs right now because there is a massive transformation going in which the fight resonance is increasing. Do not be too alarmed—this is what happens when people embrace the state of love more deeply. As the resonance of love increases, it is activating all the deadened, hardened, hidden away shells and shadows. As that frequency increases, everything that is not like love comes to the surface, similar to the way your body releases chemicals to fight a nonexistent pathogen. So there is quite a fight going on, but it simply means those hardened places are coming up for healing. Do not make the mistake of thinking that more fight will make the difference.

It is imperative, if you truly want to be a peacemaker, that you make peace with yourself. Awaken to the reality of life as it is. If you begin to feel self-righteous, pause, go inside, and notice the tension you are carrying. When you have dropped the fight and no resistance remains, love has free rein with you. As you allow that to happen, you will heal and you will become a healing force for others.

Assume that you do not know everything yet. That basic assumption will invite you to be a little more receptive to what you may be able to learn. It is hardest for people who already think they know it all. If you think you already know all the answers, there is no space for something new to arise.

Stop looking outside yourself for any explanation for the way home, or for any reason for your misery or pain or conflict. Nothing outside you is the problem or the answer. You contain within you all you need to know. You are wasting your energy when you fight or seek anything you perceive to be outside you. That is not the same as not choosing change. It simply means that your choices emanate from a space of peace rather than tension.

As you increasingly become aware of yourself as energy, you will experience your whole body as a fine vibration. This is simply a pointer. This realization of yourself does not necessarily mean you are fully awakened, but that you are recognizing yourself as dissolvable and dissolving. At that point, the surrender gets easier and the process speeds up, although what comes up then may be even more difficult to face. At least at that point you know the context within which the phenomenon is occurring. Things you held dear that you never even thought to question may dissolve. You must be willing to go there. That does not mean everything in your life will be turned inside out and upside down, but—as in Job's story—it might. You must be willing to let go of all the forms that define you. You must be willing to let go of that which is most precious to you. There is never a guarantee that you will be rescued at the last minute, although whatever you need will always be there for you.

Accepting exactly this nanosecond over and over and over again is what allows the encoding to dissolve and reform. Bit by bit, as you dissolve your old mental constructs, you will come into a sense of yourself as awareness itself.

Even the ideas you are reading here are concepts, so recognize the concepts as form and allow them, too, to dissolve. Be aware only of the breath coming and going. Surrender into the sensation of life itself pulsating in your body. Recognize every pulse as it comes and goes. The second you have a sensation in form, release it. Do not push it away, just accept. There is nothing you need to do except trust. Trust that life will present to you exactly what you need to experience at any given moment, and then let it go. When you do this, fear eventually dissolves. You will find that you *are* that life, and that there truly is *nothing* to fear!

You are never alone. That is quite a fallacy. The depth of loneliness you feel is the deep calling of your cellular structure and matrix inviting life to awaken, so go there when you feel most lonely. Dare to sit in that yearning. Invite the life that is striving to wake up right there wherever you are. Stay in the honesty of it. If you bring your awareness there, it *will* wake up—it has to. All it needs is your attention and awareness.

You are so loved. No matter how far you go, home is waiting for you. You are welcome and you are loved. Remember that. Surrender. You can do nothing that will remove you from the capability of life finding you again. Of course, you are welcome to forget that as long as you like. But the instant you remember (because there really is no time involved), you are there in the doorway. You never really left, except in your mind.

APPENDIX
Mindbody therapeutic techniques

Mindbody integration therapy stems from a different premise than conventional Western medicine in that what is valued is increased self awareness in addition to symptom relief. Patients using integrative therapies may be able to use fewer drugs and medical resources; however this is only one goal of therapy. Disease can be seen as an opportunity for exploring lifestyles, choices, and attitudes. By tuning in at deeper levels, you discover amazing things about your attitudes that may be fostering illness. Often, simply awakening to your inner self brings about the change you need to release patterns of pain and disease. Beyond relieving symptoms, pathology can be used as an entry point for increased self-awareness and understanding that will allow you to maximize your potential.

All mindbody techniques have the capacity to create the space for you to reflect deeply into yourself so you experience more clarity and understand the interaction between your physical ailments and your mental constructs. It is important for you to find both a practitioner with whom you resonate and trust, and a technique that has a fluidity and allows you to delve deeply. All techniques described in this book—and many others that you will discover as you explore what is available—can help you activate and use the healing consciousness at its most profound level. These techniques have the potential to profoundly shift your way of thinking.

Exactly how healing is accomplished varies with the technique, but certain elements consistently facilitate the process. First, the work must be consistent with the body's actual message. You constantly check in with the barometer of progress—the body. As you work together, you and your therapist are open to the story that may explain a particular experience, and you both have the willingness to discover whether recognizing the story has actually helped. This involves checking your tensions and breathing patterns on an ongoing basis. If tension remains, or the posture remains tight, the explanation is just one more intellectual tangent. Typically, the body's message is simple, such as "I'm scared," as opposed to a long, elaborate mental explanation. Remember that the story is not an end in itself, but a tool. As explored earlier, the goal is to move beyond the story. The willingness to be present in the simple space of childlike expression is one of the fulcrums of any technique's effectiveness.

One way to get in touch with the body's messages is to bring the breath and awareness to the place of tension. If you have experienced habitual tension, numbness can build up such that you "forget" what is there. Breathing deeply into this numb place can bring up these long-forgotten memories and feelings. Your therapist might place her hand(s) on tense areas, thus helping to bring your awareness to the place where the energy is stuck. This can be done with massage, acupressure, energy work, or simple touch.

Secondly, you must actually experience the stuck pattern within your feeling layer. Typically, when you and your therapist are mutually aware and that awareness is maintained in alignment with body's messages, the release of pent-up emotions happens spontaneously. This can happen as a vivid recall of an event replete with imagery or as the simple release of feelings that were never completely expressed. In either case, you are then in the best possible position for change because you have moved beyond the intellectual realm and into the experience itself. Once this happens, numerous possibilities open up. Some forms of therapy end here, with the assumption that emotionally releasing the past creates a space wherein a new reality can be developed. Sometimes this does happen. The increased clarity that comes from reliving the past in the present provides you with the needed insights to make a shift in your perceptual framework. Most often, however, it is helpful to include the third element.

This third and final element is to invite, at the level of experience, a different possibility than the one that haunts you. The key factor here is "at the level of experience." Timing and a deep respect on the part of the therapist for your inner well-being are essential. When you relive a very difficult part of your past where you felt yourself to be helpless, it is imperative that you have progressed enough to be able to perceive and experience yourself differently. This is the only way to achieve long-lasting, effective change in how you relate to your world. Allow the message for health to come up spontaneously rather than trying to force-fit a preconceived idea of what it should be. This honors your innate wisdom, which is longing to express itself.

BREATHWORK

All Western medical practitioners learned in training that sympathetically enervated functions are under the control of cognitive function and autonomically enervated functions are not. Autonomic functions include heart rate, digestive functions, blood pressure, and so forth. Actually, all of these things are influenced by mental functioning. You can gain access to them and learn to impact and change them. However, for purposes of this section, the one and only one function that is both sympathetic and autonomic is the breath. You can control the breath, but you do not need to for it to continue functioning. Like the heart, it continues unabated to keep your life going without your conscious awareness.

The breath is fundamentally important in that it continuously, breath by breath, connects the inside and the outside. In addition, it is shared from one person to another. Unlike food, which you might say connects the outside with the inside, the molecules of the air you have breathed sooner or later will be breathed by those around you, making the breath a great equalizer. It influences all functions of the body at the most profound level. It carries toxins away and brings the most basic nourishment of life into the body. In Sanskrit it is called *prana*, the life force itself.

If you pay attention to your breath, you will soon notice that, for example, if you are tense or faced with a crisis or difficulty, your breath will be altered. So if you learn to pay attention to your breath on an ongoing basis, you will very quickly notice if you are feeling anxiety. As a way of coping, you may have learned to control or ignore your own sensations, so if you pay attention to your breath you may notice when you are bothered by something—even before you "feel" bothered. By the same token, if you pay attention to your breath, you can immediately begin to alter it for positive reasons. For example, when you are feeling tense and anxious, if you do nothing more than take a deep breath you will relieve some anxiety on the spot. It may not cure the whole problem, but at least you have a handle on the situation for that moment. Sometimes that is all it takes to break the cycle. Remember, you are trying to break the momentum of mental complexity that gets you into trouble, so if you can break it soon enough, you may spare yourself considerable unnecessary grief. One day you will notice, "Hey, I was about to go into a thought pattern that would create even more trouble, but I caught myself!" It is empowering when you have that awareness. If you do nothing else beyond making a discipline of observing your breath, noticing what it is telling you, and interrupting the patterns, you will go far in your awakening process.

In addition, any time you become aware of tension in any part of your body or in a place that is holding pain, you can consciously bring your breath—at least in your imagination—to that place. This practice creates a sense of openness and spaciousness where there was tension. Often, simply by bringing the awareness of the breath into the place of pain, the pain will disappear. If it is chronic pain or tension, bringing the breath there may bring to the surface an awareness of the stuck mental construct you will need to address in a more formalized fashion. At times you may need a guide to help you with the more entrenched patterns.

The breathwork referred to in this section is not *pranayama* or other such controlled breathing techniques taught in ancient India. *Pranayamic* exercises such as "breath of fire" can increase the life force and even fairly quickly alter consciousness dramatically, and they may also have their place in your repertoire of useful techniques.

Breathwork can be used when you are in a very low energy state. Focus on the energizing quality of the breath and enter a deeply relaxed state where you allow the breath to revitalize you. This is related to *pranayamic* breathing, although you do not necessarily need to believe in that concept for it to be effective.

MEDITATION

Many techniques fall into the category of meditation. It is important to find a technique that works for you, so this section provides a general introduction to some you might be interested in exploring further. This overview is by no means fully inclusive of what is available to you.

Numerous meditative styles focus on concentrating to clear the mind. The Tibetan Buddhist tradition has many forms of meditation that involve focusing on a particular quality or virtue. These virtues are often represented by icons of certain deities that embody the desired traits. The idea is that by meditating on the deity that represents this quality or virtue, you embody the virtue within yourself. For example, to embody the sensation of love and compassion, you might choose to rest your mind on the deity Tara. Likewise, in the Christian tradition, focusing on the qualities of a particular saint can facilitate the embodiment of those virtues. In this type of meditation, you are manipulating your body's vibratory frequency, which can help to release stuck energy patterns.

Another concentration meditation is simply focusing on your breath or a mantra (a simple word or phrase). A mantra does not necessarily have to be meaningful, although some words are believed to contain a higher vibratory frequency. By focusing in such a single-pointed way, you can achieve complete concentration, allowing the distractions of your stories and other mental noise to die down. This is a very powerful practice that can take you to a blissful state.

Other forms of meditation develop the power of mindfulness, or waking up to inner processes. The practice of Zen meditation centers on noticing and accepting "what is" moment to moment. Forms of Zen meditation encompass various walking and sitting techniques. Whatever form you choose, it is important to observe what arises dispassionately, not critically. Dispassionately does not mean free of compassion, it means free of reaction.

A similar form of meditation is called *vipassana*, or mindfulness meditation. *Vipassana* is a Sanskrit word meaning "to observe." The purpose of *vipassana* is to awaken to a deeper knowing of your being. Through observing the physical structure, you begin to understand, "That which I observe is not who I am." As you simply observe sensation arising and passing away, you increasingly stop identifying with storylines and sensations. You recognize *at the experiential level* that everything in life is constantly changing, and therefore it is wasted effort to cling to anything or push anything away.

Other forms of meditation, such as the Buddhist practice of *metta*—a loving kindness meditation—take you into the compassionate heart, where you dwell in the deep knowing of compassion and love.

These different forms of meditation, and others, can be combined. You must develop both compassion and wisdom (*prajna* in Sanskrit). Meditation can help you move past your mental constructs and conditioned behaviors and open to the awareness that what flows through you is life itself. Compassion without wisdom is openness without awareness. Wisdom without compassion is sharp-edged and precise, but does not allow the safety in which to completely surrender. Compassion is the space in which wisdom can be most safely recognized. You need both to be complete, and each feeds into the other.

Remember that becoming the perfect practitioner of meditation is not the goal. The goal is to allow meditation to carry you into a deeper awareness. The peace of your meditation can go with you into every moment as you go through your day—in which case all you do is a form of meditation. It is certainly possible to remain awake and aware while maintaining activity. Let the knowing of peace—or the lack thereof—be the barometer of how much time to devote to seated meditation. Do whatever it takes to develop the ability to not get caught in the distractions. No matter which technique you use, remember that it is just a tool, not an end result. As with stories or other tools that can help us wake up to reality, it too must fall away in the end. All things eventually fall away in the awakening process.

WHAT TO EXPECT WHEN YOU BEGIN MEDITATING

As you begin meditating, you will undoubtedly encounter some common stumbling blocks. It is easy to get discouraged and give up before you really get started, so do not let that happen to you. Realize that what you are experiencing is an essential and integral part of the waking up process.

One of the first things that may happen when you quiet down in meditation is that you begin to notice bodily sensations. Being wrapped up in the busyness of your life, you may have armored and numbed yourself through self-induced anesthesia to the point you are unaware of what is going on in your mindbody. Meditation gives you enough quiet space to begin noticing whatever you have been ignoring, including bodily pain. You try to sit and cannot get comfortable. You begin to itch or feel fidgety. You notice a pain here or a pain there. And you may misinterpret what is happening, misperceiving that the meditation itself is causing you all sorts of grief. You may be tempted to run to your aspirin bottle or your physician for some medication to anesthetize yourself against it, or you may give up totally and decide you are "not the type who can meditate." It is important to remember that you are simply unmasking the first level of that which you have hidden from yourself. Instead of trying to escape, recognize the phenomenon for what it is. Become willing to sit with the physical sensations of discomfort. Become willing to see what is waiting to be revealed to you.

Another thing you will notice right away is the busyness of the mind itself. Many people become frightened or disillusioned or discouraged at this point and quit. Many people have told me, "Dr. Wallace, I can't meditate, I can't make my mind stop." And I say, "Well, if we wait until our mind stops then we will be dead, won't we?" Thinking is what your mind does. That is its job. As we go about our normal day, we hardly notice what is going on because everything moves at such a rapid pace. When you pause to allow just a tiny bit of breathing space, you can feel overwhelmed because suddenly you are aware of the magnitude and rapidity of thoughts that arise. This stream of thought has always been there, like water in the aquarium of your life. Just watch your thoughts as they come and go. You will start to notice space between the thoughts and between the body's sensations. Expand your awareness of that space within which everything occurs. Only by doing this will you gain full awareness of the fact that everything in your life, including your emotions and your thoughts, arise and pass away. When you embrace that knowing completely within the fabric of your body, you are no longer afraid. You have ultimate choice. You embrace every experience as it is, because you know it is just passing through.

Once you have been meditating for a time, you will doubtless reach a plateau or experience a time where "nothing is happening." You will become bored, and question why you are bothering. It is much easier to get up and replace that boredom with activity. Rather than cave in to this tendency, recognize how stimulation is a motivator in your life. Notice how uncomfortable it is to have periods of time free from that stimulation. Most people exist on the adrenaline rush, which they frequently feed by caffeine or other addictions. Having brief unstructured time periods can actually be quite frightening. Fear arises as you rest in the awareness of yourself as a constantly changing phenomenon. It is not an easy path. When you are called to this awareness, do not resist. Stay in your seat and watch what arises.

After you have developed the discipline to sit and observe, devoting a certain amount of time every day to this process, you may go through a period of time where you experience enormous breakthroughs that lead you to great gladness. And this may be interspersed with the struggle. Everyone's experience is different. Sooner or later, however, you may find yourself gaining a certain feeling of superiority or a perception that you now "get it." You can become lax and think you do not need to meditate anymore. This is quite a dangerous time because your mind has seduced itself completely by using meditation as the ultimate ego trip. It is very seductive. You must realize that if you are perceiving meditation as "a thing you are doing," you are still trapped in an illusion. Meditation is simply a thread in the fabric of your life experience. It can help you wake up, but it is not the awakening and it is not the goal. It is not even the path. Your body and your experience is the path. Meditation is a methodology whereby you are able to pay better attention to "what is." When you take it less seriously, you will move into a state of being in which your life is a meditation. You will no longer worry about doing it right or wrong, doing it the right amount of time, and so forth. All these concerns fall away because it is no longer something you have to succeed at. Let go of any need or pride in being the perfect meditator.

Be aware that when you begin meditating, you may experience increased aggravation around the life dilemmas you have not dealt with. This is ultimately a positive change, and is not mentioned to discourage you from doing it. Just be aware of what can happen when you begin to shift your level of awareness, and remember that your life may get messier before it gets better.

Do not let any of these stumbling blocks cause you to drop or fail to begin your meditation practice. Do find a technique that works for you. At different times in your life or on different days you may need to use a different method, so let yourself explore. Give yourself permission to learn what works for you. On certain days there may be so much ruckus going on that you may simply need to focus on your breathing to concentrate the mind. On other days you may be sluggish, so doing yoga or another movement meditation would be best. Even walking in solitude with awareness of yourself and your environment, breathing the air and noticing nature can help you get out of a rut. Just remember that it is a lifelong learning process with many phases. Make meditation a habit.

MEDITATIVE JOURNALING

Journaling is a wonderful anchoring device for meditation. When you meditate or deeply reflect, you might not later remember the insights you have gained, particularly if you are working with deeply ingrained issues to which you experience strong resistance. Recording them on the page helps to keep them in your awareness so you can consciously work with them. It is a powerful tool to help you go more deeply into the matrix of your storyline and unravel the threads.

The process consists of posing certain questions to yourself in a deeply relaxed and meditative state, then answering them—usually through a combination of writing and drawing. Although writing is the key component of the process, drawing helps to bridge the right and left brains and access the subconscious, allowing the symbols of your story to come out so you can write about them. Skill level is irrelevant to this process. You can do it even if you think you cannot draw.

Begin by equipping yourself with a notebook and plenty of colored pens, pencils, crayons, watercolors, or other writing and drawing tools that spark your creativity. An exhaustive list of ideas and questions to take into your meditation would be impossible, because the possibilities are infinite. Just allow the issues that are "up" for you to guide you to the areas you want to explore. To get started, take a few minutes to relax and become present. Pose a question to yourself, and then write or draw whatever arises. Moving from writing to drawing and back to writing can help to move deeper into the question. Find the process that works for you.

As an example of how you might use this process, try the following exercises that I use in my Meditative Journaling workshops. The first exercise will help you to examine the beliefs that underpin your basic sense of reality. As long as they remain unexamined, these

• The Heart of Healing •

beliefs drive your behavior and your life choices. Remember, the point of this exercise is not to merely replace the rules you live by with another set of rules, but to actually open to new possibilities and richer potentialities from a deeper space within you.

1. Take a few minutes to list the rules you learned from your family while growing up. These might be something like: "You should always work hard," "Never talk to strangers," or "Children should be seen and not heard." Use imperative statements such as "You should," "Never," and "Always." You may have learned these rules through direct instruction or by observing what happened around you and to you.

2. Write an overarching statement about yourself that emerges as you look at this list. For example: "I learned to be self-reliant, but at the cost of working too hard," or "I have always been safe, but I never really took any risks so my life has been pretty boring," or "I've always been a 'nice girl,' but never learned to speak my truth."

3. Make a list similar to the first one but this time, list the rules you learned from the culture at large.

4. Compare the lists and write comments to yourself about what you notice.

5. Pause. Reflect on what you might need in order to feel more whole given these messages. What would help you to feel less trapped by them?

6. Meditate. Sink deeply into the sensation of loosening the shackles of these beliefs, perhaps even freeing yourself entirely.

7. Draw any images that arise, and then write to anchor what has arisen.

8. Do this meditation daily in order to experience the new sensations associated with freedom from these old beliefs. New images will evolve spontaneously from within as you recognize the falsity of the old restrictions.

An exercise that can help if you find yourself stressing out is one I call "Worry Time." The point of this exercise is to restrict worry—usually a useless waste of energy—to a certain amount of time each day, and convert it to useful energy and action. Therefore, time yourself. Allow no more than half an hour a day to this exercise, after you have done steps 1 and 2.

1. Draw a vertical line down the center of a sheet of paper. On the left side, write down everything you are worried about. Do not leave anything out, no matter how minor it is.
2. After you have finished with your list, go back through it and write next to your worry, in the right-hand column, which things you can do something about and which things you have no control over.
3. Looking over your list, choose one of the things you can do something about. On a separate page, write the worry at the top of the page and then brainstorm what you can do about it and when. Give yourself a timeline.
4. Do the same thing with the other worries that you can do something about. Write about no more than one worry at a time during your daily "worry time." (You can add to—or subtract from!—steps 1, 2 and 3 as needed.)
5. Now choose one thing you have no control over. Meditate on that worry. Notice the sensations that arise as you allow the feelings to emerge. Stay with it until you notice the sensations changing into a sense of peaceful acceptance. Do not push it. The main thing is to remain aware and allow the sensations to change on their own. If you cannot achieve a sense of peaceful acceptance in one sitting, do the meditation daily until you are able to embrace the situation exactly as it is.
6. Do this with all of the worries you have no control over, one per day.

The point of meditative journaling is not to analyze or figure out in detail what your stories are or where they came from. It is simply to identify what the beliefs are behind the stories. The point is to wake up to the fact that you are living out your stories. From that awareness, you can see how you carry your stories in the fabric of your body, and then you can use the relaxed sensations to release the stuck energy patterns.

IMAGERY

Imagery is often referred to as visualization, but this is an incomplete description of the technique. The mind functions using all the senses, and visual images comprise just one piece of what the mind uses to construct, engage with, or perceive the world. Perhaps a third of the population never sees mental images, yet may use other senses such as hearing or tactile sensation to do imagery. Everyone is processing images at some level all the time, just beneath the surface of awareness. The rich complexes that drive our lives, including our history and belief systems, lie in the deep reservoir of our subconscious. This is where we must go if we are to evoke deep and lasting change in behaviors or patterns that trouble us.

As the word implies, imagery involves the power of the imagination to create an internal state. As early as 1929, it was discovered in the laboratory that thoughts caused appropriate muscles to twitch as if the action were really taking place. Images serve as the bridge between conscious information and physical change. It has been said, "What you can imagine you can do." What may be more accurate to say is that what you imagine fully, you already have done as far as the body memory is concerned.

Research has shown that consciously using imagery can enhance healing, promote restful sleep, increase energy, and facilitate creativity. Measurable reductions in pain, nausea, vomiting, stress, and tension have been experienced by patients using imagery. Reduced length of hospital stays and complications after surgery have been documented. Guided imagery has helped writers move through writer's block, athletes enhance their performance, and patients heal by activating the immune system. By holding—with feeling—certain images, you can affect your heart rate, blood pressure, immune function, blood glucose levels, and muscular tension.

Engaging in imagery as a therapeutic regimen is not using something artificial or unusual. It is simply awakening to what was there to start with, and using it for your benefit. Awakening to the imagery that is going on in your mind *all the time* can become a profound spiritual tool. Noticing your physiologic response will lead you to those mental constructs that engage the mind, and is an invaluable awakening tool.

TYPES OF IMAGERY

There are basically three types of imagery: guided imagery, interactive imagery, and healing imagery. **Guided imagery** involves harnessing the imagination to move your consciousness in the direction you want it to go. It is a method whereby all senses are engaged in the imagination to invoke certain states. It usually begins with deep relaxation and then images are introduced that will, for example, facilitate sleep, increase creativity, or reduce pain. Guided imagery is usually done using a skilled coach or listening to a prerecorded tape or CD. The therapist will invite you into a scenario that is meant to precipitate in the body exactly those physiologic responses that are desired. Once a sequence is memorized, however, it is relatively easy for you to involve your imagination on your own. You induce the desired state, such as relaxation or alertness, by imagining certain scenes or repeating certain phrases. It is a form of self-hypnosis.

If I said to you, "Reduce your blood pressure," it is unlikely that it would happen. But what if, on the other hand, I said to you, "Imagine your breath coming in easily and deeply. As you take a deep breath, you suddenly find yourself walking on the warm sand of a beach with the sun touching your cheek. With another breath, you can smell the salt air and feel the breeze wafting across your forehead, tousling your hair a little. You begin to notice every step. You are barefoot now, and the sand is warm…." As you amble along the beach in your mind's eye, a surreptitious blood pressure check would undoubtedly demonstrate that it has lowered. The imagery has just profoundly affected your autonomic nervous system.

As another example, imagine that you are late to an important meeting with your boss or a major client or that you are on your way to your daughter's championship soccer game with her in the car.

You are stopped at a railroad intersection with a train going by. As the minutes and the train cars pass, you are getting later and later. You begin to notice certain physiologic effects. Your blood pressure is going up, your heart rate increases, your palms sweat, and you are gripping the steering wheel. Perhaps your neck muscles are tensing up and you are beginning to get a day's worth of headache. But you are just sitting in your parked car! It is all going on inside your head, and it is acutely affecting your physiologic response. Learning to consciously use imagery to counteract these conditioned responses can make a significant difference in your ability to remain calm and balanced when faced with life's challenges, and this in turn will have a more positive affect on your physiology.

Interactive imagery can include guided imagery, but goes a step further. By increasing your awareness of what is contained in the mindbody, interactive imagery allows you to communicate at a much deeper level. It brings you to a deep state of internal awareness within which you can find and interact with problematic, "stuck" images. Your internal portfolio sets you up to either block or to facilitate goals you set for yourself. By engaging at this level, you deal with the scripts that are getting in the way. For example, you might get help with interactive imagery to uncover inner resistance to success or to explore the roots of recurring conflict.

Let's say you have no clue why your arm is hurting. You have discovered by deepening your awareness that the more you pay attention to it, the more it hurts. This is a perfect opportunity to consciously use imagery as an interactive tool. Ask questions of your arm. Believe me, it will answer you—sometimes in words, but more likely in a felt sense. For example, sooner or later you may awaken to the fact that the job situation in which you exist day after day is not the best for you. You may or may not have known that, but you probably didn't realize the profound effect it was having on your body without stopping long enough to pay attention.

Not long ago, a patient who had done a fair amount of doctor shopping came to see me with chronic back pain. He attributed his pain to having sustained a work-related accident years before. In taking his history, I ascertained a fair amount of contained anger, and it seemed clear to me that he had some issue with authority. A brief query uncovered a difficult relationship with his father. In this case, I used a combination of interactive imagery and acupressure, so I was able to feel the tension in his back. After inducing deep relaxation, the pain in his back completely vanished. He expressed his astonishment at this and I, as a small test, invited him to remember the conversation with his father he had mentioned earlier in the session. His back immediately went into spasm such that he jumped while on the table. In that moment, he was able to see the intense connection between his contained anger, the back pain, and the angst he had in relationship with his father and other authority figures. The connection he made that day was an important step toward healing and helped him to understand the need for deeper therapy around those issues.

Using imagery does not necessarily tell you what you need to do about what you discover, but awakening to the fact that you are in a situation that does not enhance your life or fulfill your potential is an important noticing. In this way, you can use your body as the biofeedback mechanism to tell you when it is time to look deeper into an issue. As discussed throughout this book, the mental constructs laid down as neurological hard wiring have created whatever situation is playing out in your life, and the first step in gaining access to those constructs involves waking up to what your body is telling you. It involves asking the hard questions. Interactive imagery is an extremely useful tool to accomplish this goal.

Using a combination of interactive and guided imagery is profoundly powerful in the healing process. Having a good guide to help with **healing imagery** is recommended, because for healing imagery to work, you need to access in an interactive way the deeper parts of the mind where the blocks to healing reside. This typically is not the area of mundane everyday thought, but requires deeper access. Introducing imagery over the top of deeper internal beliefs without first ferreting out those beliefs can create wonderful feelings and get you through a crisis, but tends to be a temporary change unless you also interactively deal with the inner dialogue. As we have explored, in order to truly heal you must account for, accommodate, and even bless all aspects of yourself—including the difficult places. Especially the difficult places.

GOAL OF IMAGERY THERAPIES

The ultimate aim of using imagery is to get beneath all your images and recognize them for what they are, not just replace the images that have caught you in their painful grip. Please remember you are still writing stories—you are just writing a more pleasant one for the time being. Do not get caught in the trap of thinking that now you have created the "right" storyline for your life. Your new storyline may create more comfort, but mostly it serves you best as a method whereby you wake up to the recognition that is simply a story.

Even a beautiful story is not who you are. It may be comforting for a while, but it is not who you are. Who you are is infinity, a point of awareness in an infinite sea of consciousness, and it is constantly changing. Getting caught in any story or role or script is a trap that sets you up for failure, because sooner or later it will change and then you run the risk of losing your sense of identify, which is what causes your suffering. Do not remain attached to anything so temporary, because that is precisely what leads you back to the fight/protect mentality.

DREAMWORK

Unresolved mental constructs have been unconsciously driving your behavior all your life, but they are so familiar or obtuse you do not notice. You tend not to recognize the roles you are playing. Often these mental constructs needing your attention come to you as dreams. Dreaming accesses the subconscious in a direct, symbolic way, and the energies in the body can be quite magnified in the dream state. The neuronal pathways are still firing even as you are sleeping, and they intrude upon your awareness such that you remember them in pictorial form.

The parts of ourselves that are unfamiliar or uncomfortable are contained in the subconscious pool from which dreams come. By working with dreams in an integrative way, you are assimilating those parts of yourself you have discarded or not yet learned about. Dreamwork can be an easy way to deal with mental constructs because you are less likely to make the error of thinking the problem is outside you when you are dealing with your own dream inside your own head. Effective dream techniques are those that actively engage the process of the dreamer. Beyond interpreting the "meaning" of a dream, dreamwork is the pragmatic application of its content.

The first step in dreamwork is recall. If you have difficulty remembering dreams, there are several helpful things you can do. First, take your dreams seriously. View them as direct forms of communication from you to you. Second, keep a journal and pen or a tape recorder near your bed so you can easily record dreams during the night. Do not expect to remember all your dreams. Unless you recognize a dream for least three minutes in beta awareness, which is your fully awake state, it is unlikely that you will recall it in the morning. However, recording even dream fragments can often suffice to bring the full details into memory.

Another technique for increasing dream recall is to set an alarm to awaken yourself a few minutes before your usual wakeup time. You become accustomed to a cyclic rhythm of dreaming, and if you come fully into beta awareness while in the dream state, you can remember your dreams more easily.

Lastly, because we usually roll over just prior to awakening, if a dream is hazy, try rolling back over. You will not remember having been in this position, but it can make remembering your dream easier. Then take the time to relax back into the inner space of dreamland. It almost never helps dream recall to struggle by willpower to force the memory into awareness.

Once you have a recorded dream, there are many ways to work with it. You might want to work with an informed therapist, but you can certainly do this on your own. One simple technique is to assume the position of each of the characters in the dream as if that character were you. Write it all out like a script, or remember it clearly. In so doing, back away from it as if you were describing a play. Notice the scene and the roles each character is playing. See if you can describe the dynamic in such a way that it might be narrowed down into a theme or statement of belief.

For example, Tom had a recurring dream in which he had a need to catch an airplane, but he had no ride to get to the airport. This dream occurred nightly for a week. The phrase he distilled from his dream was, "I need to do something that I am unable to do." Once you have distilled your dream into a statement, rest deeply in your body and feel the sensations that arise when you hold that thought in your mind. It is helpful to reinsert yourself into the dream and recognize the neuronal pattern that is playing out in your body. Rest assured that you have just revealed a theme song for your life at that particular moment in time. In Tom's case, upon reflection he was able to recognize that the statement he uncovered by scripting his dream reflected a theme he has dealt with his entire life. He is nearing the end of his life, so his subconscious has invited him to squarely face this huge burden.

When you go into the sensations of your body, recognize that whatever you feel is simply a habit. Recognize it as a pattern, not a reality. Embrace yourself having that experience. If you want to, you can change the storyline long enough to imagine what it might feel like to easily choose a different ending for the dream. For instance, Tom might visualize that he gets a ride to the airport. This only works if you really experience it in your body. The point is not necessarily to change the story, but to wake up to the fact that the story is fluid and you *can* change it. You can own the story; do not let the story own you. If you are experiencing a recurring theme in your life, your story owns you. So if you decide to play with rewriting the story, recognize it as a crutch. You do not require a new story to live by; you must simply recognize that it is all a story and you can find new ways of relating to it.

Dreamwork can also be done in a group with an informed group leader. You can assign different group members to play a particular part in your dream and give instructions as to how they are to feel, behave, and interact. Do not try to rigidly control them, but do help them to get the dynamics straight. As they play the parts of your dream, observe the sensations in your body as you watch the script play out. Really experience the internal impact this action has on you. If you want, you can stop the scene, recognize how you would like it to be different, rewrite the script, and let them play out the new script. Again, pay attention to the sensations in your body. Notice how your sensations may be different as you see the script written differently and the storyline resolved in a different way. Remember, the point is to wake up to the fact that it is all a story and the story is fluid, so you can rewrite it anytime.

By entering fully into the dream's dynamic from the unique position of each character in turn, you will more fully understand your own complexity. All characters, their activities and interrelationships, and the scenario come from within you. By observing closely, you are privy to your own internal drama. Each of us is composed of many parts, and many of those parts may have differing opinions and agendas. These parts can conflict, and internal wars are waged at the level of our subconscious. By revealing your internal patterns to yourself, you gift yourself with the possibility of change. Once you have conscious awareness of these internal characters' tendencies, you can make choices—as those characters—to do something differently.

When you do this work, you may begin to notice when the script appears in your waking life, and how fluid the story really is. Recognize the different choices available to you. You will notice the ways the dynamic plays out, and soon you will catch yourself in the middle of a reaction or a script. You will recognize it as a script and recognize that you have complete freedom to react in new ways.

Dreamwork is a powerful way to wake up to your scripts. People ask me sometimes, "Dr. Wallace, are you sure it isn't just the pizza I ate?", and my answer is always no—even if the pizza *was* the physical stimulus. There are no mistakes. We invite into our lives the stimuli that will facilitate our awakening. That is a guarantee.

WORKING WITH THE ENERGY BODY

Ancient practices like meridian therapy, acupuncture, acupressure, qigong, tai chi, and other modalities have been used for thousands of years to manipulate the energy body. Because they facilitate energy flow, they are extremely helpful. Likewise, Ayurvedic medicine springs from a culture that recognizes the body as energy and as part of the environment in which it exists, reflecting an awareness that we cannot get to by dissecting the body. These healing methods can help to prevent many maladies, and those who practice them can live longer and sometimes appear youthful right up to death. Working with the energy body definitely holds value beyond simply manipulating the biology allopathically, and if these teachings were included in basic Western medical training, it would provide a far advanced method of treating the body.

However, while it is useful to think of the human body as pure energy, it is important to recognize that who you really are ultimately is beyond energy. Energy is the interface—the rapidly dancing atoms. It is matter, and you are more than matter. Matter is finite, and you are infinite. Although awareness of the energetic state increases the fluidity of change, recognize that you are still dealing with the three-dimensional world. The energy body is not necessarily ongoing after what you call death, so do not be confused about that.

ENDNOTES

[1] Most religions tell some version of the story about the "fall of man" and "original sin." Throughout this book, I refer to version of the story told in the Judeo-Christian tradition. I offer this synopsis here not because I believe it is factually true, but because I believe it is metaphorically and metaphysically true. From this viewpoint, the story can teach us much about the human condition. As told in Genesis 2:4-3:24 in New International Version of the Bible, God creates the Garden of Eden and places Adam there to care for it. In the center of the garden are the "tree of life" and the "tree of knowledge of good and evil." God commands Adam not to eat of the fruit of the tree of knowledge or he will die. He then creates Eve as a helper for Adam, and they live in the garden naked and unashamed. A serpent comes along and convinces Eve that she will not die if she eats the fruit of the tree, but instead she will be like God, knowing good and evil. She eats the fruit and gives it to Adam, who also eats. When God comes looking for them, they hide because they are afraid he will see their nakedness. God curses Adam and Eve, condemning them to a life of suffering, saying "The man has now become like one of us, knowing good and evil. He must not be allowed to reach out his hand and also take from the tree of life and eat and live forever." He gives them "garments of skin" and banishes them from the garden, placing cherubim and a flaming sword at the entrance to guard the way to the tree of life.

[2] Again referring to a story from the Book of Job in the Christian Bible, Job's story is one of complete faith in the face of unspeakable trials. As God's faithful servant, Job is blessed with great wealth and many children. Then one day, all is taken from him. His livestock and servants are stolen or killed, his children die tragically, and he is inflected with

painful sores from head to foot. Although his faith is severely tested, he remains true to God, and in the end his steadfastness is rewarded. God restores his health, doubles his wealth, and gives him many more children and a long, happy life.

[3] Vipassana meditation is one of India's most ancient techniques of meditation. Meaning "to see things as they really are", it involves scanning the bodymind with the intention of nongrasping awareness in order to awaken to the knowing that all things are impermanent. This can lead to enlightenment.

[4] Maslow was one of the early psychologists who focused his theories on studying individuals who had achieved psychological health. He developed a hierarchy of needs, beginning with the basic physiologic needs (hunger, thirst, fatigue), through safety needs (avoidance of pain, anxiety; desire for security), belongingness and love needs (affection, intimacy, need to have roots in family or peer group), esteem needs (self respect, adequacy, mastery, competence) to the need for self-actualization (to be fully what one can be).

[5] Chakras refer to seven main energy centers or "wheels" in the body. According to ancient Hindu literature, each chakra is concerned with specific aspects of human development and behavior. They are:

1) the root chakra located at the base of the spine which relates to basic survival needs
2) the spleen chakra located just above the genital area which relates to sexual energy and basic interpersonal relationships
3) the navel chakra located at the umbilicus which relates to raw emotion, power drives and social identification
4) the heart chakra located at the level of the heart which relates to love, compassion and goodwill
5) the throat chakra located at the front of the throat, which relates to self expression
6) the brow chakra (or "third eye") located between the eyebrows which relates to clear sight of the truth and heightened self awareness

7) the crown chakra located on the top of the head which relates to the experience of self-realization or enlightenment.

[6] From the Mahayana tradition of Buddhism, a *bodhisattva* is an enlightened being who continues to incarnate, putting aside his or her own final enlightenment in order to help others achieve enlightenment.

ABOUT THE AUTHOR

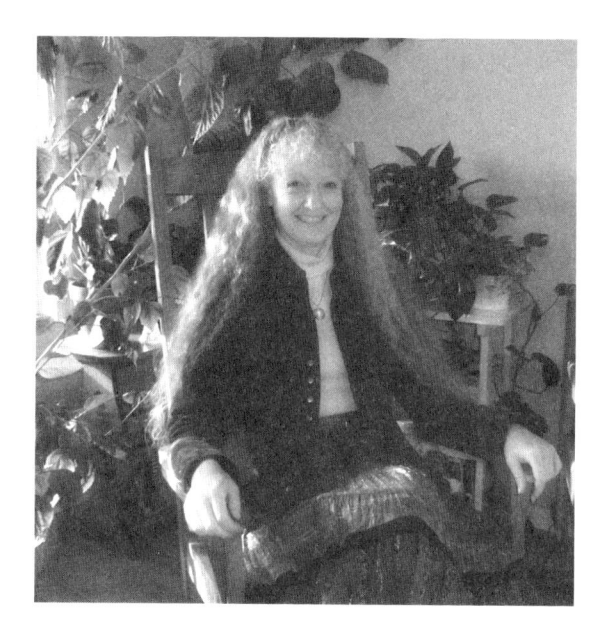

$\mathcal{D}$r. Mary Ann Wallace is a board-certified physician specializing in internal medicine. As a pioneer in the field of mindbody medicine, she has extensive training and experience with numerous holistic healing modalities, including meditation, breathwork, imagery, dreamwork, acupressure, process-oriented psychology, vision quests, therapeutic touch, and herbology.

Dr. Wallace serves as medical director for an expanding, self-sustaining integrative medicine program within a large metropolitan hospital system. As a leader who focuses on empowering others, Dr. Wallace takes a uniquely spiritual approach to classic problems such as conflict resolution, building trust, communication skills, and relationships.

For nearly 30 years, Dr. Wallace has led workshops and classes on spirituality in medicine and mindbody issues. She is an accomplished and engaging speaker who has given more than 400 lectures on complementary/alternative/integrative medicine to medical professionals and laypeople. She is frequently invited as a keynote speaker at conferences.

In her presentations and workshops, Dr. Wallace integrates meditative mindfulness, warmth, humor, and scientific data—all informed by decades of experience. She offers a rare opportunity for healing and transformation in a safe and supportive environment. Several of her presentations are distributed on CD and videotape.

"When Dr. Wallace speaks to a group she is always very warmly received. She really seems to hit the pulse of where we're trying to bring the group. She can get people so focused immediately in that moment. It's totally amazing to work with her and it doesn't matter if it's a small group of people, if it's a group of four or five, or if it's a roomful of people, she is just a phenomenal presence. Every time she walks into a room there's just this peaceful presence around her. She's so authentic— I think that's the best word. You always feel like you are the most important person when you're talking to her."

Dawn M. Fucillo, MA, RT, (T) (QM), CMD
Director, Regional Cancer Center and Mario Pastega House
Samaritan Regional Cancer Center, Corvallis, Oregon

To order books, CDs or for information on workshops and services offered by Dr. Wallace, see www.maryannwallace.com.